HEADACHE

HEADACHE

Understanding, Alleviation

JAMES W. LANCE

CHARLES SCRIBNER'S SONS, NEW YORK

Library of Congress Cataloging in Publication Data

Lance, James W
  Headache: understanding and alleviation.

  Bibliography: p.
  Includes index.
  1. Headache. 2. Analgesics. I. Title.
RB128.L34   616'.047   75-11809
ISBN 0-684-14372-0

1 3 5 7 9 11 13 15 17 19 H/C 20 18 16 14 12 10 8 6 4 2

Printed in the United States of America

Contents

Acknowledgments

I am deeply indebted to my secretary, Mrs. R. M. Kendall, for her constant help and meticulous attention to detail in the preparation of the manuscript. The figures were drawn by Mrs. F. Rubiu and photographed by the Department of Medical Illustration, University of New South Wales, Sydney.

I am grateful to William Collins & Co. Ltd., London, for permission to quote from James Jones's *The Icecream Headache and Other Stories;* to Robert Hale, London, for permission to quote from Ward McNally's book *Smithy: The Kingsford Smith Story;* to W. B. Saunders and Co., Philadelphia, for permission to quote from *Psychosomatic Medicine* by E. Weiss and O. S. English (3rd Ed., 1957); and to News Limited, Sydney, for permission to use the cartoon on pp. 102–3 from *The Australian* of October 25, 1974. Some of the material presented in this book is based on my earlier book for medical readership, *The Mechanism and Management of Headache,* London, Butterworths, second edition, 1973.

It is impossible to acknowledge adequately my debt to my colleagues in neurology and other branches of medicine in many parts of the world whose ideas have influenced those expressed in this book. Truly we all see further by standing on the shoulders of those who have gone before.

Introduction

This book has been written for the person who has no medical training but who wishes to know something about one of mankind's oldest problems and what is being done about it. It is not intended to act as a self-diagnosis kit but does provide a guide to the causes and treatment of headache. The secret of headache management is collaboration between patient and doctor. The object is to abolish headache completely, or at least to reduce it to the point where it no longer interferes with the enjoyment of life.

Most people have experienced a headache at some time in their lives. Those who haven't are inclined to think that headaches are a refuge of the escapist or neurotic. They may think differently after reading this book. There must be very few who are not confronted with the reality of headache among family, friends, or colleagues.

The relationship between a doctor and his patient has changed gradually over the years and continues to change. In the days when the level of education in the community was not very high and medical knowledge only marginally higher, it was sufficient for the physician to make a pronouncement and supply a bottle of medicine to keep most of his patients content. Nowadays patients are more curious, more critical, and better informed and want to understand the basis of medical disorders so that they can cooperate in treatment. It is not unusual for the question to be asked casually at the end of a consultation, "By the way, what is the cause of migraine?" The question can be answered, but it takes more time than the last few minutes of an interview.

It is hoped that this book will answer many such questions. If it proves interesting as well and helps some patients rid themselves of headache, it will have fulfilled its purpose.

1
Ten Thousand Years of Headache

The common forms of headache are thought of as the by-product of a frenetic industrial age, the wages of stress. Yet neurological colleagues from countries where the pace has scarcely quickened in a thousand years assure me that headache complaints are often heard in the local dialect, where there is a doctor ready to hear them. I have seen women working in the rice paddies of Java with cloth bands tied around their foreheads. These were not designed to keep the sweat from their eyes, as I had supposed, but were "headache bands," a traditional remedy for headache. Dr. Reuben Taureka, now Minister for Education in Papua-New Guinea, told me that it is a common practice for tribes in the highlands to scarify their foreheads because of recurrent headaches.

In primitive Melanesian communities on islands of the South Pacific, the custom of trepanning persisted until recently. (Trepanning is an operation in which a hole is made in the skull with some sharp implement in order to let out evil spirits.) The Melanesians used trepanning as a treatment for insanity, epilepsy, and persistent headache. Skulls showing signs of trepanning have been found in Europe and on the American continent, particularly Mexico and Peru, dating back to the Neolithic and Bronze ages. The openings in the European skulls were mostly oval, and the edges showed signs of healing, indicating that the operation had been carried out during life and that the patient had survived for some time afterward. If we can accept these trepanned skulls as evidence, the history of headache extends back ten thousand years or more, and we can picture Stone Age man clutching his shaggy brow to appease the demon within it.

Even if we limit ourselves to written accounts, headache still has a history of respectable antiquity. The earliest medical records of many great cultures make reference to it. Headache is mentioned in the *Atharvaveda* of India, a book on the knowledge of magic formulas gathered between 1500 and 800 B.C.

Our knowledge of medicine in Egypt comes from two papyri named after their discoverers. The Edwin Smith Papyrus, written in about 1700 B.C., was based on earlier writings dating back to 3000–2500 B.C. It describes the appearance of the brain and the types of paralysis which may follow injury to the head. The Ebers Papyrus, written about 1600 B.C., also contains fragments which originated one thousand or more years earlier. One extract reads, "List of the virtues of ricinus [castor oil plant]: it was found in an ancient book concerning the things beneficial to mankind. If its peel is brayed in water and applied to a head that suffers, it will be cured immediately, as though it had never suffered."

From the Babylonian era, we have an interesting and poetic reference to headache which probably dates from 4000–3000 B.C.

Headache roameth over the desert, blowing like the wind,
Flashing like lightning, it is loosed above and below;
It cutteth off him who feareth not his god like a reed,
Like a stalk of henna it slitteth his thews.
It wasteth the flesh of him who hath no protecting
    goddess,
Flashing like a heavenly star, it cometh like the dew;
It standeth hostile against the wayfarer, scorching him like
    the day,

This man it hath struck and
Like one with heart disease he staggereth,
Like one bereft of reason he is broken,
Like that which has been cast into the fire he is
    shrivelled,
Like a wild ass . . . his eyes are full of cloud,
On himself he feedeth, bound in death;
Headache whose course like the dread windstorm
    none knoweth,
None knoweth its full time or its bond.

An extraordinary case report from Hebrew medicine is to be found in the Bible (2 Kings IV: 19–20): "And he said unto his father, my head, my head. And he said to a lad, carry him to his mother. And when he had taken him, and brought him to his mother, he sat on her knees till noon, and then died." However this is not the end of the story of this serious, apparently fatal, headache. The prophet Elisha was summoned, and as he was approaching he was met with the news that "there was neither voice, nor hearing . . . the child is not awaked." Elisha "went up, and lay upon the child, and put his mouth upon his mouth . . . and the flesh of the child waxed warm . . . the child sneezed seven times, and the child opened his eyes." The sudden onset of headache, followed by loss of consciousness with recovery after mouth-to-mouth resuscitation provides a dramatic description of a life-threatening headache of intracranial origin, possibly caused by a form of cerebral hemorrhage or encephalitis.

Greek medicine really starts with Aesculapius who may have lived about 1250 B.C. So successful was his medical practice that Pluto became concerned because the supply of souls to the Underworld was dwindling and requested Zeus to remove Aesculapius from the register of doctors, which Zeus promptly did, with a thunderbolt. After his death, Aesculapius became re-

garded as a god, and temples dedicated to his name
sprang up throughout Greece. These temples, known
as Asklepieia, were devoted to healing the sick. The
sick would sleep in the colonnades at the side of the
temple so that they might be visited by Aesculapius,
given advice, and cured. Some of the miraculous cures
were recorded on stone tablets. One tablet at Epidaurus describes how Agestratos (classified as case number
29) suffered from insomnia on account of headaches. As
soon as he came to the temple he fell asleep and had a
dream. He thought that the god cured him of his headache and, making him stand up, taught him wrestling.
When day came he departed cured, and after a short
time he competed at the Nemean games and was victor
in wrestling. The cure was not remarkable since no
failures were recorded on any of the stone tablets.

The scientific age of medicine began with Hippocrates, who was born on the island of Cos in 460 B.C. and
was said to be a direct descendant of Aesculapius. His
fame rests largely on his meticulous observation of disease and his recording of details of his patients, including his failures as well as his successes. He formulated
an ethical code of conduct for physicians which persists
in principle to this day. He described a headache which
was probably migrainous:

> Most of the time he seemed to see something shining
> before him like a light, usually in part of the right eye;
> at the end of a moment, a violent pain supervened in
> the right temple, then in all the head and neck, where
> the head is attached to the spine . . . vomiting, when it
> became possible, was able to divert the pain and render
> it more moderate.

A detailed description of migraine was given by
Aretaeus, a physician who was born in Cappadocia in

Asia Minor, now part of Turkey, about A.D. 81 and who practiced in Alexandria. He emphasized the fact that the pain commonly affects one-half of the head, which he called heterocrania.

> In certain cases, the parts on the right side, or those on the left solely, so far that a separate temple, or ear, or one eyebrow, or one eye, or the nose which divides the face into two equal parts; and the pain does not pass this limit, but remains in the half of the head. This is called heterocrania, an illness by no means mild, even though it intermits, and although it appears to be slight. For if at any time it set in acutely, it occasions unseemly and dreadful symptoms, spasm and distortion of the countenance takes place; the eyes either fixed intently like horns, or they are rolled inwardly to this side or to that; vertigo, deep-seated pain of the eyes as far as the meninges; irrestrainable sweat; sudden pain of the tendons, as of one striking with a club; nausea, vomiting of bilious matters; collapse of the patient . . . there is much torpor, heaviness of the head, anxiety and ennui. For they flee the light; the darkness soothes their disease: nor can they bear readily to look upon or hear anything agreeable; their sense of smell is vitiated, neither does anything agreeable to smell delight them, and they have also an aversion to fetid things: the patients, moreover, are weary of life, and wish to die.

Galen (A.D. 131–200) later called one-sided headache hemicrania, which is the origin of the Old English *megrim* and the French word *migraine* which is now in common use.

In A.D. 600, Paul of Aegina, a Greek physician at the Medical School of Alexandria, wrote, "Headache, which is one of the most serious complaints, is sometimes occasioned by an intemperament solely; sometimes by a redundance of humours, and sometimes by

both." This carries on the views originating in early
Greek medicine, and confirmed by Galen, of four humors which governed health and disease—blood,
phlegm, yellow bile, and black bile. This was transmuted over the centuries to four "temperaments"—
sanguine, phlegmatic, melancholic, and choleric—
words we still use. In the present day, a humoral agent
is a substance carried by the blood which can influence
remote parts of the body by chemical means, a process
which is now considered to play an important role in
the mechanism of migraine. We could bring Paul of
Aegina's penetrating observation up to date by saying,
"Headache is sometimes the result solely of nervous
tension, is sometimes brought about by humoral agents,
and in some both factors may play a part."

Thomas Willis (1621–75), a London physician, wrote
one of the first textbooks on the anatomy of the brain,
Cerebri Anatome, which was illustrated by Christopher
Wren, the architect of St. Paul's Cathedral. He divided
habitual headaches into those which were continuous
and those which were intermittent, a distinction which
remains of fundamental importance today. In Willis's
case book, written in 1683, he reports the case history
of a noble lady with migraine which has often been
quoted and deserves reproducing once more.

> Some twenty years since, I was sent for to visit a most
> noble lady, for above twenty years sick with an almost
> continual headache, at first intermitting: she was of a
> most beautiful form, and a great wit, so that she was
> skilled in the liberal arts, and in all forms of literature,
> beyond the condition of her sex, and as if it were
> thought too much by nature, for her to enjoy so great
> endowments without some detriment, she was ex-
> tremely punished with this disease. Growing well of a
> feavour before she was twelve years old, she became

obnoxious to pains in the head, which were wont to arise, sometimes of their own accord, and more often upon every light occasion. This sickness being limited to no one place of the head, troubled her sometimes on one side, sometimes on the other, and often thorow the whole compass of the head. During the fit (which rarely ended under a day and a night's space, and often held for two, three or four days) she was impatient of light, speaking, noise or any motion, sitting upright in her bed, the chamber made dark, she would talk to no body, nor take any sleep, or sustinance. At length about the declination of the fit, she was wont to lye down with a heavy and disturbed sleep, from which awaking she found herself better, and so by degrees grew well, and continued indifferently well till the time of the intermission. Formerly, the fits came not but occasionally, and seldom under 20 days of a month, but afterwards they came more often: and lately she was seldom free. Moreover, upon sundry occasions, or evident causes (such as the change of the air, or the year, the great aspects of the sun and moon, violent passions, and errors of diet) she was more cruelly tormented with them. But although this distemper, most grievously afflicting this noble lady, above 20 years (when I saw her) having pitched its tents near the confines of the brain, had so long beseiged its regal tower, yet it had not taken it: for the sick lady, being free from a vertigo, swimming in the head, convulsive distempers, and any soporiferous symptom, found the chief faculties of her soul sound enough.

He concludes on a pessimistic note regarding her response to treatment.

There was no kind of medicines both cephalics, antiscorbuticks, hysterical, all famous specificks, which she took not, both from the learned and the unlearned, from quacks, and old women, and yet notwithstanding

she professed, that she had received from no remedy,
or method of curing, any thing of cure or ease, but that
the contumacious and rebellious disease, refused to be
tamed, being deaf to the charms of every medicine.

The nineteenth century brought in the Golden Age
of description and classification in medicine, although
it must be said that therapy remained in the age of
baser metals. The first major work concerned solely
with headache was Edward Liveing's book, *On Me-*
grim, sick-headache, and some allied disorders: a con-
tribution to the pathology of nerve storms, published in
1873.

Primitive medicine, which is still in use in some countries, draws on a rich drug lore based on native plants
and combines this with charms, incantations, or witch-
craft, a powerful psychological support. In a ritual used
by the Cherokee medicine man·for the treatment of
headache, the patient chews ginseng, the root of a plant
with medicinal properties, while the forehead is
rubbed gently with the palm of the right hand as the
medicine man sings:

The men have just passed by, they have caused relief,
The wizards have just passed by, they have caused relief,
Relief has just been rubbed, they have caused relief,
    Sharp!

The medicine man then blows water mixed with ginseng juice on the painful area. The whole ceremony
could be repeated up to four times if necessary.

Acupuncture has been used in traditional Chinese
medicine since it was devised by Huang Ti, who was
said to have lived from 2698 to 2598 B.C. It is said to
puncture the twelve hypothetical invisible channels
which contain the Yang, the active male element, and
the Yin, the passive female element, restoring the bal-

ance between them. Because of recent reports of its efficacy in relieving headache and other pain, acupuncture is being studied by modern scientific methods.

It is only recently that the investigation of the pathophysiology of headache has begun in earnest and that its treatment has assumed some scientific basis. The general use of aspirin preceded the knowledge that it blocked the action of substances which play a part in inflammatory processes including headache. The new era was ushered in by the pioneer work of Sir George Pickering in London during the 1930s on the headache produced by histamine, and by the painstaking studies of the late Dr. Harold G. Wolff and his colleagues in New York covering almost every aspect of the problem, culminating in Wolff's book *Headache and Other Head Pains* which is the modern classic on the subject. Some of the work currently in progress in different parts of the world will be described later in this book. It would be impossible to name all those who have contributed and are contributing to knowledge at the moment. Among them are Arnold Friedman, formerly of New York, and John Graham of Boston, Donald Dalessio, the members of the American Association for the Study of Headache who have carried on the Wolff tradition in the United States, and Federigo Sicuteri, who has developed a headache center in Florence, Italy, which has provided a source of original ideas for the past fifteen years. Other groups in Britain, Scandinavia, continental Europe, and our own team in Australia continue the search for the complete understanding and cure of migraine and other forms of headache. W. G. and M. A. Lennox in their book *Epilepsy and Related Disorders* recount a delightful anecdote which is a fitting conclusion to this brief historical survey of ten thousand years of headache.

About once a month, until the age of 70, George Bernard Shaw suffered a devastating headache which
lasted for a day. One afternoon, after recovering from
an attack, he was introduced to Nansen and asked the
famous Arctic explorer whether he had ever discovered
a headache cure.

"No," said Nansen with a look of amazement.

"Have you ever tried to find a cure for headaches?"

"No."

"Well, that is a most astonishing thing!" exclaimed
Shaw, "You have spent your life in trying to discover
the North Pole, which nobody on earth cares tuppence
about, and you have never attempted to discover a cure
for the headache, which every living person is crying
aloud for."

2
Why Does the Head Ache?

Headache is a constant or pulsating pain felt in the head. Why do we feel pain at all? Pain is normally a protective device for the body so that any threat of damage can be avoided. If we prick ourselves on a sharp object, we withdraw our hand or foot from it. If we sprain an ankle, pain forces us to rest the joint until it recovers. Pain is caused by impulses that pass along the nerve fibers, like brief electrical discharges. Most nerves in the body can give rise to the sensation of pain if the frequency of discharges within the nerve fibers increases rapidly. For example, touching a warm object with the hand will set up a train of impulses in the nerves passing from the hand to the spinal cord. As the object becomes hotter, the number of impulses each second increases. If heat becomes so great that the skin is in danger of being burned, the nerve fires off impulses rapidly and continuously. This burst of activity is then interpreted by the central nervous system as pain.

Some nerve fibers specialize in conveying the message of pain. One group conducts the impulses quite quickly and another very slowly. If we touch a hot stove, we remove our hand immediately because of a sharp painful sensation. A second or so later another throb of pain is felt as the slower nerve fibers deliver their message to reinforce the first.

The sensation of pain thus serves a useful purpose. It is only when it becomes excessive and persistent that it ceases to be a warning device and becomes an agent of misery. Pain in the head can arise from the nerve fibers responsible for sensation in the scalp, muscles, and bones of the neck and skull. More commonly it comes from arteries which supply the face, scalp, and brain with blood because the arterial walls contain fine nerve filaments, called a nerve plexus, which are highly sensitive to stretch.

I have heard an occasional person boast that he or she has never experienced a headache and does not know what headache is; at the other end of the scale are those unfortunate people who react to commonplace situations by developing a headache. Others are subject to headache without any discernible reason in their life or their surroundings.

Headache is almost entirely subjective. Doctors have to rely on the description of the person who suffers from it to make a diagnosis and assess its severity. For this reason we cannot tell whether animals suffer from headache. It is true that a very severe headache will cause pallor, sweating, nausea, and vomiting but mostly the observer has little else to guide him than the subject's own words. Even though everyone lives in his or her own perceptual world, the perception of pain does not differ greatly from person to person.

PAIN THRESHOLD

The pain threshold can be measured by a number of standard methods, such as the application of measured amounts of heat to the skin. This threshold has been found to be remarkably consistent, varying for one person only 3 percent from the average value and within a group of two hundred people by no more than 15 percent. It appears from all experiments that the pain threshold in humans is fairly stable and bears no consistent relation to age, sex, fatigue, and the normal range of emotions. The threshold is lowered by a previous injury to a particular area or by sunburning of the skin and can be raised by hypnosis, suggestion, distracting the attention, concentration on other things, and by competing stimuli such as acupuncture.

Medications which relieve pain, known as analgesics, can also raise the pain threshold, but so can dummy tablets. Hippocrates pointed out that "of two pains occurring together, not in the same part of the body, the stronger weakens the other." This is the principle of counterirritation as illustrated in the use of linaments to relieve limb pains or by the application of hot cups, which produce a partial vacuum as they cool, to the chest. This traditional treatment for pleurisy is still in vogue in some parts of the world.

While the sensation of pain is much the same in everyone, the reactions to it differ widely. Some of these reactions are reflex and usually not subject to voluntary control, such as alteration of heart rate, blood pressure, and the blood supply to the skin which controls skin color. When headache is present, there is often a reflex contraction of the muscles of the head and neck which may give a feeling of stiffness to the neck. Other physical reactions, which are under voluntary control, depend upon the cultural background and upbringing of the individual. Some people are much given to expression of their bodily sensations in colorful language and gesticulation. Others may have a more stoic philosophy, and their symptoms can then be uncovered only by careful questioning. Those who are interested and active in the world around them may suppress the sensation of a mild headache and carry out a normal day's routine. Others who lead a solitary life and are inactive, depressed, or introspective may dwell on their symptoms until their severity becomes progressively magnified. Fear walks hand in hand with pain. If a patient does not understand that a headache is typical of migraine or nervous tension, he or she may be afraid that it is caused by a cerebral tumor or that it could lead to a stroke. The idea of such a disaster grows in the mind until he or she can think of little else. Explaining the causes of pain and the natural history of the headache is thus the first step in coming to terms with the symptoms and helping to overcome them. The more a person understands the cause of his or her headache, the more calm and relaxed he or she becomes, and the more the intensity of the headache is reduced. The less pain that is experienced, the more the headache is seen in perspective to the rest of life, and the process of relaxation is thus reinforced. What could have been a vicious circle—pain and anxiety spiraling upward together—is converted to a gentle decline of symptoms, with pain and anxiety ultimately subsiding together.

PAIN PATHWAYS

Pain from the head and neck comes from the nerves supplying the skin, scalp, muscles, and joints or from the deeper structures, such as the skull and the membranes lining the brain. Curiously enough the brain itself is insensitive to pain. In fact, some brain operations can be carried out with the patient wide awake. If the surface of the brain, the cortex, is touched or stimulated by an electric current, the patient may feel a tingling down the opposite side of the body, see flashes of light in front of the eyes, or experience other sensations depending upon the part of the brain which is stimulated. But the patient does not feel pain even if the brain tissue is cut with a scalpel.

The largest of the nerves, which is responsible for

sensation from the face and for the front two-thirds of the scalp, is called the trigeminal nerve because it has three separate divisions (Figure 1). (The Latin *trigeminus* means "three born at a birth.") If this nerve is irritated it causes pain in the forehead, cheek, or jaw, depending on which of the three divisions is involved. If, for example, sinuses in the forehead are inflamed, the swollen lining of the sinuses compresses the fine nerve branches embedded there. The pressure sets up nerve impulses which travel along the first division of the trigeminal nerve. If the maxillary sinuses (antrums) in the cheek bones or a tooth in the upper jaw become infected, pain is conveyed by the second division. If a tooth in the lower jaw or the jawbone itself is the cause of the trouble, the pain impulses travel in the third division. The three divisions join together inside the skull where their combined fibers enter the brain-stem, which lies under the brain like the stalk of a mushroom (see Figure 1). Some fibers pass directly upward into the brain itself while others make a loop downward into the upper part of the spinal cord. This loop is of great importance in the understanding of pain in the head and neck because it connects with the same nerve cells that receive impulses from the upper part of the neck. For this reason, a disturbance of the bones or disks in the upper part of the head and neck can cause pain to be felt in the eye and forehead, a phenomenon known as referred pain. When this pathway is operating in the reverse direction, a headache such as migraine can be accompanied by severe pain and stiffness in the neck.

In addition to supplying the face and skull with pain sensation, the trigeminal nerve is responsible for sensations coming from the blood vessels in the brain and scalp. The commonest sources of headache are dilatation, distension, and displacement of the blood vessels.

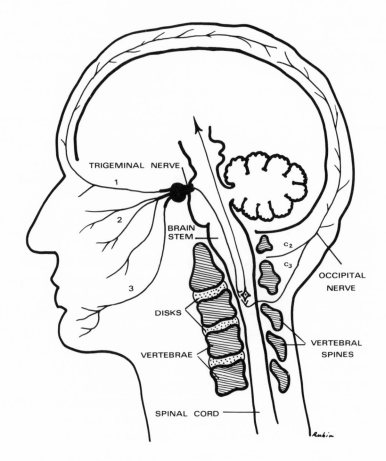

Figure 1. Main nerves of the head.   Sensation from the front part
of the head, the cheek, and the chin is conveyed by the three
divisions of the trigeminal nerve (numbered 1, 2, 3). Sensation from
the back part of the head travels in the occipital nerves through the
second and third cervical spinal nerve roots (labeled C_2, C_3). Some
nerve fibers of both pathways connect with the same cells in the
upper part of the spinal cord, thus allowing pain arising from the
neck to be felt in the forehead and vice versa.

When an artery becomes distended, the delicate network of nerve fibers around it stretches and gives off signals which may increase with each pulse, so the headache may be described as throbbing. The arteries of the scalp are mainly responsible for some forms of headache like migraine, and can be felt to be pulsating more than usual. Firm pressure over the pulse in front of the ear or over the affected area will diminish the severity of the headache because less blood flows through the sensitive vessels with each pulse. In other forms of headache, such as hangover, the arteries inside the skull are dilated and sensitive so that jarring of the head or bending the head forward will make the pain worse.

If we draw a line straight upward from the ear, any pain in front of that line results from activity in the trigeminal nerve, and any pain behind the line comes from the spinal nerves which run down over the back of the head to join the upper part of the spinal cord. The same spinal nerves supply the lining of the rear of the brain and the brain-stem so that pain felt in the back of the head can arise from inside the skull or from the upper part of the neck. These principles can be illustrated by some kinds of headache which are not symptoms of any serious disease but can occur in most people under certain circumstances.

"NORMAL" HEADACHES

The nerves we have been discussing respond to touch, pressure, heat, and cold as well as pain. If any of these stimuli becomes excessive, the increasing number of impulses generated in the nerves signals the sensation of pain. Even wearing a tight hat will give rise to pain after a while. Diving into very cold water can cause a sudden headache. Eating very cold food can excite the nerves in the mouth and palate to cause headache. This has been called "ice-cream headache" and is another example of referred pain because branches of the trigeminal nerve supply the areas inside the mouth as well as the head.

ICE-CREAM HEADACHE

Holding ice or ice cream in the mouth or swallowing it while it is still very cold may cause a localized pain in the palate or throat and sometimes a headache in the forehead or temple because of referred pain from the trigeminal nerve endings. Occasionally it may produce pain behind the ear because this area is supplied by another cranial nerve, the glossopharyngeal, which also has branches over the back of the throat that may be thrown into sudden activity by intense cold. The condition is sufficiently well known to have been used as a title for a collection of short stories, *The Ice-Cream Headache* by James Jones. In the title story, referring to the grandfather and the grandchildren, Jones wrote, "He loved to feed them large doses of ice cream on summer afternoons, would laugh at them gently when they got the terrible sharp headaches from eating too much too fast, and then give them a gentle lecture on gluttony."

The condition was mentioned as far back as 1850 in Daniel Drake's *Principal Diseases of North America*.

> The consumption of ice cream has been increasing in the Valley, for the last quarter of a century; previously to which its use was quite limited. At present, it is used in summer, in all our cities, from the Lakes to the Gulf of Mexico; and makes an important part of the luxuries

provided by the wealthier classes, for their evening parties, throughout the year. For a long time, many persons regarded it as dangerous in hot, and absurd in cold weather; but these prejudices are now nearly extinct. I have not had occasion to observe any injurious effects from it, that might not be traced to two heads: first, swallowing it before the ice has dissolved in the mouth, when it sometimes raises an acute pain in the pharynx, and gives a sense of coldness and sinking in the stomach; second, eating it when the stomach is torpid and inactive from dyspepsia, and the individual is inclined, at the time, to sick headache. The composition, not less than the coldness, contributes to the injury in this case. Under all other circumstances, ice cream may be regarded as equally salubrious and pleasant.

The origin of ice-cream headache is sudden cooling of the roof of the mouth. Cooling of the esophagus (the tube which connects the throat with the stomach), or of the stomach itself, does not cause headache.

Other forms of headache result from simple dilatation of the blood vessels inside the skull, particularly the intracranial arteries. Continuing the gastronomic line of thought, we can now consider headaches caused by certain foods or chemical substances contained within them. We shall leave the question of foods triggering migraine headache to a later chapter.

HOT-DOG HEADACHE

Some individuals develop headache shortly after eating hot dogs or other cured meat foods. Originally rock salt was used in the preparation of cured meats. The patchy appearance of the final product was caused by sodium nitrite, an impurity of the salt. Nitrites are now added to salt in order to produce a uniform red look to the meat. Nitrites are well known as dilators of blood vessels and, even though the usual concentration of nitrites in cooked meat is only 50 to 130 parts per million, some people are susceptible to headache after eating hot dogs, bacon, ham, or salami.

Doctors William R. Henderson and Neil H. Raskin of San Francisco studied a man who experienced a moderately severe headache in both temples within thirty minutes of eating cured-meat products. The attacks usually lasted for several hours, sometimes accompanied by flushing of the face. The man did not have headaches at other times. It was found that small amounts (10 milligrams) of a solution of sodium nitrite produced a headache for this man eight out of thirteen times while a solution of sodium bicarbonate of similar taste and appearance had no effect. This particular patient was also sensitive to tyramine, another chemical which will be mentioned later in the chapter on migraine. Normal volunteers did not react to either chemical substance.

THE CHINESE RESTAURANT SYNDROME

Some unfortunate people experience sensations of pressure and tightness in the face, burning over the trunk, neck, and shoulders, and a pressing pain in the chest after eating a Chinese meal. A few of them also complain of headache—usually those who are susceptible to migraine or other vascular headaches. The headache is a pressure or throbbing over the temples and a bandlike sensation around the forehead, coming on twenty to twenty-five minutes after eating Chinese food and lasting for an hour. Doctor Herbert H. Schaumburg and his colleagues in New York have shown that the offending substance is monosodium

L-glutamate (MSG) which is widely used as a food additive, particularly in Chinese cuisine. All subjects tested developed the "Chinese restaurant syndrome" if they consumed enough MSG on an empty stomach. Once some other food had been eaten, even the most susceptible did not develop headache. For this reason, soup usually precipitated the headache as it is consumed before any other food is taken. About three grams of MSG will produce an attack in sensitive individuals. This amount is contained in about 200 milliliters (seven ounces) of wonton soup. The symptoms are caused by the direct action of MSG on blood vessels. Moral: take food before soup in a Chinese restaurant if you are one of the unhappy few.

HANGOVER

MSG is not the only dilator of blood vessels. Alcohol is a potent dilator as the flushed appearance of any bon vivant will testify. In addition, some wines contain histamine, a potent dilator in its own right. Patients who are prone to migraine may notice that red wines trigger off a migraine attack, but that they can drink white wines without any worry. The histamine content of alcoholic drinks, particularly red wine, is sufficient to trigger off attacks of migraine and cluster headaches in some patients and may add to the effects of alcohol in the well-known hangover headache. The histamine content of various alcoholic drinks is shown in the following table:

HISTAMINE CONTENT (milligrams/liter) OF WINES
AND OTHER ALCOHOLIC DRINKS

Wines	White	Red	Investigator
French	0.19	14.6–15.6	Granerus, Svensson, and Wetterquist, 1969
German (Moselle)	0.04		Granerus, Svensson and Wetterquist, 1969
Italian (Chianti)		2.5–2.8	Granerus, Svensson, and Wetterquist, 1969
Californian	0.3–11.4	0.3–15.5	Ough, 1971
Australian	0–0.7	1.1–3.0	
			Trewethie, 1972
Spanish Sherry		2.0–2.9	Granerus, Svensson, and Wetterquist, 1969
Port		0.05	Granerus, Svensson and Wetterquist, 1969
California Sherry		0.6–3.1	Ough, 1971
Champagne		0.3–1.9	Ough, 1971
Swedish, Danish Beer		0.3–1.5	Granerus, Svensson, and Wetterquist, 1969
Brandy		0	Granerus, Svensson, and Wetterquist, 1969
Scotch Whiskey		0	Granerus, Svensson, and Wetterquist, 1969

I have been unable to obtain figures for bourbon, gin, or vodka, but it is unlikely that histamine would be found in any distilled drinks.

Since a hangover is usually a feature of the morning after, it is probably not the direct result of alcohol but rather the effect of its breakdown products (acetaldehyde and acetate) which are then circulating in the blood and cause a painful relaxation of the arteries inside the skull. The added factors of a late night, loud conversation or music, excitement, and possibly nervous tension and cigarette smoking may all contribute to the end result. Remedies which constrict blood vessels, including caffeine in coffee and tea, are helpful, as well as the usual analgesics.

FASTING HEADACHE

While excess of some foods and drinks can touch off headache, abstaining from food may do the same in some cases. Lowering of the blood sugar level is a known trigger for migraine, and a dull headache often accompanies any prolonged fast. The chain of events is complex and appears to involve the formation and release of fatty acids into the blood stream. Just because a headache regularly occurs in the early hours of the morning, it does not mean that it is caused by a low blood sugar. And it is not likely to be prevented by eating before going to bed.

REBOUND HEADACHE

Substances such as caffeine, nicotine, and ergotamine constrict blood vessels and therefore diminish any vascular headache. If these substances are continually entering the blood stream, the vessels adapt to a semiconstricted state and they will dilate, causing headache, if the constricting agent is withdrawn. The sufferer from tension headache who habitually takes caffeine in tablets or powders of A.P.C. (aspirin, phenacetin, and caffeine) may develop a headache as the effect of the tablets wears off. Similarly, a consistently large amount of tea or coffee can lead to a withdrawal headache if the supply is not maintained. Patients who have been pre-

scribed ergotamine to ward off a migraine attack are ill
advised to take these pills every day. If they do, the
chances are that they will prevent one headache only
to lay the foundation for the next. This type of headache is called "rebound headache" because of the cycle
of vascular constriction and dilatation. It is probable
that smokers' headaches belong in the same category
because of the constricting effect of nicotine, although
nervous tension may also be partly responsible.

EXERTIONAL VASCULAR HEADACHES

Now that we have shown that food, alcohol, tea, coffee,
and smoking can all play a role in provoking headaches,
it seems only fair to incriminate sporting and sexual
activities as well. It can be seen that avoidance of all
activities which have been known to cause headache
can lead to a fairly quiet and unadventurous existence.
There is no need to lose heart, however, because these
forms of headache are not very common and can be
prevented in ways other than a monastic life.

Any form of exercise can precipitate headache in
some unfortunate people. One young man was on the
verge of giving up competitive sports because he invariably developed a throbbing headache after strenuous exertion. Another patient was unable to finish a
day's work in his garden because of headache. In both
cases the headache could be prevented by taking tablets to constrict the blood vessels of the head before
starting the day's exertion. Exercise can also provoke a
migraine headache in some cases, and this may be prevented in the same way. During exercise, the blood
pressure rises, the pulse rate increases, and arteries
throughout the body increase in diameter. This process
of dilatation normally affects the small vessels as well as
the large so that the face becomes flushed and veins

stand out on the temple or forehead, indicating that blood is flowing more rapidly through the scalp. The probable cause of headache during exercise is that the smaller vessels do not dilate enough to keep pace with the larger ones, and the face remains pale even though the arteries are distended and pulsating more than usual. The blood in the arteries is under increased pressure because it cannot escape easily through the small channels in skin and muscle. The vessel wall is therefore stretched and gives rise to the sensation of pain. The treatment, which ensures that the arteries do not dilate excessively, is to give ergotamine tartrate or methysergide before beginning exercise or to use other agents to flush the skin and relax the small vessels (these act as valves preventing the free flow of blood through the dilated arteries). Another possibility, which may appeal to some, is to give up exercise.

COUGH HEADACHE

A variation on exertional vascular headache is a headache felt only on coughing, sneezing, bending, or straining. Sometimes this may be a serious symptom because it can happen when there is some obstruction of flow through the normal fluid channels of the brain, the ventricles. It always warrants a consultation with a doctor. It used to be thought that coughing headache was invariably due to a serious cause until Sir Charles Symonds, a great English neurologist, described twenty-seven patients with coughing headache of whom only six were found to have a brain tumor or similar intracranial abnormality. He coined the term "benign cough headache" to describe the symptom of the remaining twenty-one patients because fifteen of them gradually improved without any treatment. Doctor E. D. Rooke of the Mayo Clinic studied 103 patients who complained of headache on running, bending, coughing, sneezing, lifting, or straining when they have a bowel movement. This form of headache was more common in men than in women in a proportion of 4:1. After ten years had elapsed, seventy-three patients had lost their headaches entirely or had greatly improved. In only ten patients was any structural abnormality found during the follow-up period. The outlook is therefore good, but it is important that the patient remain under the supervision of a neurologist, who will ensure that the condition is indeed "benign cough headache."

SEXUAL INTERCOURSE HEADACHE (BENIGN SEX HEADACHE)

Headache occurring at or near the climax of sexual intercourse is happily uncommon. It may be intensely severe, throbbing or bursting in character and naturally gives rise to much alarm and apprehension. It is true that the increase in blood pressure which accompanies enthusiastic sexual intercourse may sometimes be of serious import if there is some underlying abnormality in the blood vessels of the brain. In some cases it is simply the result of muscle contraction and a sudden dilatation of the blood vessels in response to an increase in blood pressure. I wonder if Hippocrates had this in mind when he wrote of "immoderate venery" in the fifth century B.C., "One should be able to recognise those who have headache from gymnastic exercises, or running, or walking, or hunting or any other unseasonable labour, *or from immoderate venery.*"

The late Harold G. Wolff described four patients, all women, aged forty to fifty-six, who experienced sudden severe pain in the head at the beginning of orgasm. The headache lasted from several minutes to several days in different instances. In one patient in whom the headache persisted, the opportunity arose to record the blood pressure, which was found to be high. After the blood pressure had subsided and the headache had disappeared, the patient became emotionally upset. Her blood pressure again shot up and the same type of headache recurred. It is well known that sudden increases of blood pressure from other causes may also provoke a transient vascular headache.

Over the years I have seen occasional patients with this form of headache and have made careful notes of five who were examined in the last two years. Three were men and two were women, all between twenty-four and fifty-seven years of age. The headache involved the back of the head only, "like a cramp," in two but spread over the whole head as an intensively severe bursting or throbbing sensation in the others. Two of the patients commented particularly that the headache pulsated with each heart beat, and two others were conscious of a particularly forceful beating of the heart at the same time. In two of the men the headache came on at the time of ejaculation and lasted only a few minutes in one, but continued for five to six hours in the other. The third man gave a clear description of the headache starting as he approached climax. If he then stopped sexual activity, the headache subsided in five to ten minutes, but if he proceeded to climax, the headache became intensely severe and persisted for up to twenty-four hours. Headache in the two women lasted for only five minutes, coming on with orgasm in one and on "striving toward orgasm" in the other. The headaches were definitely not related to the amount of physical exertion during intercourse. Only one of the five had noticed any form of headache on exercise at other times. Others played vigorous sports such as tennis or squash without ever developing headaches. One man had analyzed his symptoms carefully with a variety of techniques. He found that the headache came on just as severely if he lay on his back and was caressed by his wife without any physical exertion at all on his part. However, he was aware of intense contraction of the jaw and frontal muscles as he approached orgasm and said that he was quite unable to relax.

The headache appeared to be related to two factors, muscular contraction and emotional excitement. Two had noticed similar but milder headaches in situations of nervous tension, and one found that he could prevent the onset of headache during sexual intercourse by deliberately relaxing his neck and facial muscles. Emotional excitement is probably the most important factor because of increasing blood pressure and causing the release of epinephrine and norepinephrine. It is of great interest that one patient had experienced a similar headache on another occasion after taking a tablet of pseudephedrine which has an effect on the heart and blood pressure similar to epinephrine.

Masters and Johnson gave physiological data taken from their studies of the human sexual response which support the views expressed concerning the mechanism of the two components of headache. During orgasm, the heart rate increases to 110 to 180 beats per minute and blood pressure rises by 20 to 80 percent. The cardiovascular changes are just as great during masturbation as in sexual intercourse. Masters and Johnson also comment on muscular contraction which they call "myotonia." They state "with plateau phase established, myotonic response is clinically obvious from forehead to toes of the responding individual. In reacting to elevated sexual tension levels, the individual frowns, scowls or grimaces as facial muscles contract involuntarily in semispasm." "During automanipulation the jaws frequently are clenched spastically."

Again, "The muscles of the neck contract involuntarily in a spastic pattern. As the result, the neck is usually held rigidly in mid-position." It is quite clear that the muscle contraction described is sufficient to initiate the greatest tension headache of all time.

Doctors G. W. Paulson of Ohio and J. L. Klawans, Jr., of Chicago recently described fourteen patients with this condition which they called "benign orgasmic cephalgia." They noted that eleven of their patients had experienced migraine headache in the past, but this did not apply to my patients. It remains a mystery as to why the condition should suddenly start to occur at a particular time, not related to the age of the patient. It warrants keeping an eye on the patient's blood pressure, but it otherwise seems to be a completely harmless condition which might vanish as suddenly as it appeared. It is possible that it may be prevented by taking certain pills before sexual activity starts such as ergotamine tartrate (used in the treatment of migraine) or agents which prevent the action of epinephrine. However, it is so unpredictable, occurring on some occasions and not others, that a pharmacological approach hardly seems worthwhile. The term "benign orgasmic cephalgia" seems appropriate although I would prefer to call it "benign sex headache" in line with "benign cough headache" and similar entities.

Enough has been said to show that a headache may arise in anyone when the nerve supply to the blood vessels or other structures of the head is stimulated excessively. It is important to be sure that these headaches are simply an overreaction of normal structures to unusual circumstances and do not indicate any abnormality of these structures or their nerve pathways. The physician is fortunately able to give that reassurance to most of the patients who consult him or her.

3

Headache from the Nerves, Not a "Nervous Headache"

When people say that a headache is caused by "nerves," they usually mean a state of anxiety or nervous tension. This will form the subject of a later chapter on muscle contraction headache, often called tension headache. Other types of headache are more literally produced by direct irritation or compression of the nerves supplying the head, face, or neck.

A nerve contains many fibers, most of which are enclosed in an insulating wrapping called a myelin sheath, like wires inside a cable. Each group of fibers comes from a particular area of the body and is responsible for sensation in that area. It is said to "supply" the area so that we speak about the nerve supply to the forehead, cheek, or chin, referring to branches of the trigeminal nerve which convey sensation from those parts of the face to the central nervous system. The nerves bring information into the spinal cord where it is transmitted to other nerve cells and pathways relaying it to the brain.

A nerve conveys its message in responding to any stimulus by setting up an electrical discharge. The electrical discharge or "impulse" passes along the nerve as a signal to the spinal cord. The interweaving of nerve pathways in the spinal cord and brain has much in common with electrical and electronic circuits so that the term "nerve circuits" is often used to describe them.

When a nerve is compressed anywhere along its course, pain may be felt to arise at the point of compression. More often it is felt as though it comes from the whole area supplied by that nerve. If, for example, a sinus infection is irritating a nerve deep inside the cheekbone, an ache may be felt not only in the cheek but also in the upper gum and teeth which are supplied by branches of the same nerve. The site of pain may be further complicated by two different nerves plugging into the same central circuit within the spinal cord or brain. Some of the central fibers concerned with the perception of pain from the forehead loop downward in the brain-stem and make connections with the same cells as spinal nerves which enter the cord in the upper part of the neck (Figure 1). This may lead to a misinterpretation of the origin of pain. A disk in the upper part of the neck pressing on one of the roots of the spinal nerves can cause pain not only in the neck and back of the head but also in the forehead. This is called "referred pain" and is caused by the curious economy of nature in making two nerve pathways converge on a single pathway.

The type of pain set up by an abnormality in a nerve or its central connections, called neuralgia, may be jabbing or persistent. Since the trigeminal nerve is responsible for sensations of the face and the front part of the scalp, we can start by considering pain arising from it.

TRIGEMINAL NEURALGIA (TIC DOULOUREUX)

Any pain originating from the trigeminal nerve may properly be called trigeminal neuralgia, and yet the term is usually applied to a particular type of pain, distinctive and devastating, which strikes its victim like lightning. Unlike lightning, it strikes the same place more than once, again and again, until its repeated jabs may drive the patient to despair. Its name is tic doulou-

reux, French for "painful spasm," an understatement
hallowed by several centuries of usage.

Tic douloureux affects women twice as often as men
and most commonly starts after the age of forty. The
pain is caused by a change in the pattern of impulses in
the trigeminal nerve. Instead of the nerve carrying a
regular pattern signaling a touch on the face, it fires off
a synchronized barrage of impulses which send an inappropriate signal of sudden pain. The pain is often triggered off by touching a particular part of the face, or
even by wind blowing on the face. It may be brought
on by talking, chewing, brushing the teeth, or shaving.
The pain most commonly strikes the gum, cheek, or
chin as a sudden stab or repetitive stabs, although in
about 5 percent of cases the forehead may be affected.
The important characteristics of the pain are its severe
intensity, its brevity, and its tendency to recur in cycles.
There may be spontaneous remissions for months or
years before the symptoms return.

What is the cause of this nerve becoming hyperexcit-
able on one side of the face? There is still controversy
as to whether it is simply the result of an age change in
the nerve cells or whether there is some subtle compression of the nerve fibers in the majority of cases.
Doctor Frederick Kerr of the Mayo Clinic thought that
the nerve might be affected by pulsation in the internal
carotid artery which lies directly beneath it in the floor
of the skull. Doctor Peter Jannetta, when Professor of
Neurosurgery at the University of Pittsburgh, reported
his experience of operating on patients with tic douloureux aged from twenty-eight to seventy-nine years, using a binocular microscope to examine the nerve where
it enters the brain-stem, an area not seen in conventional operations performed to cut the nerve. Of the
first one hundred patients, ninety-four were found to
have some identifiable source of compression or irrita-

tion of the nerve fibers. The most common cause was a branch of an artery which had progressively lengthened as it hardened with age until it touched on the nerve. Doctor Jannetta reported that most of the patients in whom he moved the artery away from the nerve later lost their pain. This operation involves a major surgical exploration of the brain-stem.

There are some patients in whom compression of the nerve can be suspected clinically because a constant pain persists between the jabs, or part of the face may feel numb or peculiar. In 2 to 3 percent of patients with multiple sclerosis, a condition in which the insulating myelin sheaths around nerve fibers break down in the central nervous system, tic douloureux may occur as a symptom.

In the majority of patients no signs can be found on examination or special tests to show any structural abnormality. The question then arises about the best way to treat the pain. Before treatment is started, it is worthwhile having a dental examination because the pain may be aggravated if the bite is uneven and throws strain on one side of the jaw.

Brain cells fire off synchronously in epilepsy in a manner rather similar to trigeminal nerve cells in tic douloureux. For this reason, antiepileptic drugs are now being used in the treatment of tic douloureux with considerable success. Carbamazepine (Tegretol) is the medication most often prescribed and may keep the pain under control indefinitely, but the treatment does mean taking pills regularly. If pain continues, branches of the nerve or the nerve itself may be injected with alcohol to deaden the area or stop the pain. This is usually a temporary measure, and pain recurs after a year or so. The nerve can then be injected again or a brain operation can be undertaken to sever appropriate divisions of the nerve or to examine it for any source of compression. If the nerve is cut, part of the face will feel numb permanently, so that it may be advisable to inject the nerve first so that the patient may experience temporary numbness and thus know what to expect.

GLOSSOPHARYNGEAL NEURALGIA

This condition is one hundred times less common than trigeminal neuralgia. It affects the nerve which supplies sensation to the back of the tongue and throat and also a nearby nerve, the vagus, a branch of which supplies the ear. It has a similar jabbing quality to tic douloureux, but the pain stabs the ear and the back of the throat on the same side and is triggered off by talking, swallowing, or coughing. The treatment follows the same principles as that for tic douloureux.

NEURALGIA AFTER SHINGLES (POSTHERPETIC NEURALGIA)

The word "shingles" comes from the Latin *cingulum* meaning a belt or girdle. The condition is an infection of a nerve root, and the resulting blotchy red rash and blisters usually run around half the body like a belt. Shingles may also affect the trigeminal nerve, usually as a band extending over one side of the forehead. Since the condition may be painful, it comes into consideration as a cause of headache. It is caused by a herpes virus called herpes zoster; hence the name postherpetic neuralgia. The virus is the same as the one causing chicken pox, and the disease probably represents a reinfection of the body by this virus in later years. It is not to be confused with the virus herpes simplex which causes the common cold sore on the face.

After the rash of shingles subsides, it leaves in its wake a partially numb area which may ache. The virus infection alters the normal composition of fibers in the nerve so that the usual pattern of nerve impulses is out of balance and may be interpreted as pain. The changes caused by the virus extend into the central nervous system since cutting the affected nerve does not always relieve pain. Recently, cortisone has been given in the active phase of the illness to ease pain and prevent the neuralgia which may follow the illness. This treatment carries a slight risk of spreading the infection, thus producing an attack of chicken pox. It has not had any more serious reactions in people who were otherwise well. Once the pain is established it can be treated by local measures, such as the use of vibrators over the affected area or repeated intravenous infusions of a dilute solution of a local anesthetic, which often gives some lasting benefit. Some pills that elevate the mood of the patient, such as amitriptyline, also have an action on central nerve pathways and diminish the pain. Radiotherapy to the affected nerve roots has been said to stop the pain, but I have no personal experience with this.

OTHER NEURALGIAS

The word "neuralgia" is overused and is often applied to any persistent pain in the head or face. Disorders affecting the skull bones may set up neuralgic pains and so may problems with the teeth, sinuses, and other nearby structures. Many of the conditions described in the older medical literature as neuralgia are now known to be variations of migraine and are therefore called facial migraine, or "lower-half headache," or are known to be a form of cluster headache.

One very strange kind of neuralgia has been designated "atypical facial pain" because it is not typical of any of the known causes and its origin is unknown.

The pain is usually felt in the angle of the nose, the upper gum, and the cheek. It is constant and penetrating in quality and fluctuates in intensity with the patient's mood, being barely noticeable when the individual is occupied and happy and scarcely tolerable when the patient is introspective and miserable. So closely is the pain bound up with the emotions that it has been regarded as a symptom of a depressive state. This explanation is not entirely satisfactory because the pain persists, at least in some measure, even when the person concerned is relieved of any associated depression. It is common experience that the condition is not improved by operations on the teeth, nose, or sinuses or by blocking the various nerves which contribute to the perception of pain from the affected area. Although the face becomes numb, the pain continues. It may be relieved by antidepressant pills, so that the patient can live with the disorder. Electric shock therapy has been reported to cause improvement. The operation of leucotomy, which divides the nerve pathways in the brain with those centers in the frontal lobe responsible for emotional appreciation, will enable a patient to tolerate the pain more readily but will not completely remove it. The essential factor for any form of treatment is missing: knowledge of the site of origin of the pain. I suspect that it will be found in the central connections of the second division of the trigeminal nerve, but the condition is a rare one and most surgeons are reluctant to perform an exploratory brain operation for a condition which has been considered to exist in the mind rather than in an identifiable part of the brain.

PAIN FROM THE EYE

When anyone develops headaches, almost invariably someone suggests the possibility of eyestrain, and a consultation with an eye doctor follows. What is eyestrain? The term means that the patient needs glasses or has an imbalance of the eye muscles which requires a continual effort to overcome. Imbalance of the eye muscles means that the eyes tend to drift inward or outward unless the individual concentrates on keeping the visual axes parallel. We are all familiar with the feeling of seeing double when we are tired. The print blurs and then separates into two images. With a conscious effort we can bring the images together again. Some people have to make this effort all the time to keep the eyes aligned. The muscular activity required for this may set up a headache. The problem may be helped by eye exercises.

More severe pains can arise from the eye if the pressure within the eyeball increases (as in glaucoma) or if there is pressure on the eye from a tumor in the eye socket. Some forms of glaucoma may be mistaken for migraine because pain is felt in the eye, radiating over the forehead on that side. This can easily be checked by an ophthalmologist measuring the pressure in the eyeball.

SINUSITIS

There is no mistaking a fully blown attack of acute sinusitis. The nostril is blocked on one or both sides and pain extends over the cheek or forehead. The affected area is tender if it is tapped with the finger, and jolting or jarring it gives rise to pain. The sinuses are air cells present in the bone of the forehead (frontal sinuses) and in the cheek bone on each side (maxillary sinus or antrum), while others are situated deeply behind the bridge of the nose (sphenoid and ethmoid sinuses). The sinuses are filled with air, and their secretions drain freely into the nose. They are responsible for the normal resonance of the voice. If the mucous membrane lining the nose swells, the small openings of the sinuses become blocked, and their secretions are retained. The voice becomes dead and lifeless without its usual timbre, as it does when we have a cold in the nose. If the patient is subject to any changes in air pressure when the sinus opening is blocked, a severe pain may be felt in the forehead or cheek. Anyone who has had this experience when traveling by air will make sure that in future he carries a nasal decongestant spray with him to cope with this painful emergency.

The treatment of sinusitis requires that the airway in the nostrils be established again by shrinking the mucous membrane with decongestant drops or spray. It is best to lie on a bed with the head tilted back so that the drops run to the back of the nose where the opening of the sinuses lies. Once the nostril is clear, the patient sits up and bends forward, and the nose can be blown once more to try to clear the retained secretions. A good old-fashioned steam inhalation is often helpful, followed by an application of dry heat attained by sitting in front of a radiator or infrared lamp. Pills containing ephedrine or pseudephedrine can be taken two or three times during the day to help constrict the blood vessels of the mucous membranes. If the sinuses are severely infected, antibiotics are given as well, but they cannot replace the free drainage of the sinuses into the nostrils. If free drainage cannot be achieved, the sinus may have to be pierced under local anesthetic by an ear, nose, and throat surgeon to form a new opening. In these days of antibiotic therapy, there are still occasional instances of sinusitis or ear infections which have not been treated adequately and infection can spread to the cranial bones or even the brain. Fortunately, most cases are cured rapidly and completely.

Sinusitis may be present in disguise in a situation which does not suggest any possibility of infection. For example, I have seen a number of patients who have developed over the preceding few days a one-sided headache, radiating backward over the head from the forehead, without any temperature or nasal blockage. Because the headache was made worse by head movement or jolting, both patient and doctor have naturally become concerned. Under these circumstances radiology can give the answer, and an X ray may show one or both frontal sinuses to be full of fluid. One of my patients complained of a constant pain in the center of the forehead which had been increasing over the past week, again without any nasal symptoms. X rays showed the region normally occupied by the sphenoid sinus, which is tucked away deeply in the center of the skull bones, to be opaque. At first the radiologist was skeptical and thought that the sinus might have been absent from birth in that particular patient, but when the X rays were retaken after the sinusitis had been treated and the headache had been relieved, they showed that this sinus was indeed present and had cleared completely.

Some patients are said to awaken with a "vacuum headache" if the opening in the sinus is blocked and the air in the sinus is absorbed, leaving a negative pressure inside. This is comparable to the more severe headaches encountered by air travelers experiencing rapid changes in altitude. Various types of pain around the eye and forehead have been ascribed to deviation of

the bone plate (nasal septum) which separates the nostrils or to enlargement of one of the horizontal bones
which divide into layers the air stream flowing through
the nose. I remain dubious about the nasal origin of
most of these pains. I remember attending a meeting
where a surgeon stated that he had cured ninety-seven
out of one hundred patients of headache by operating
on the nose. One of his colleagues whispered to me how
extraordinary it was that the only three patients in
whom the operation was unsuccessful must have been
the ones that he himself had referred to that surgeon
since none of the three had benefited at all from the
procedure. The evaluation of surgical or any other
treatment of headache must be very carefully compared with the results of other treatments and with the
known course of the untreated illness. Headache often
improves spontaneously. If the doctor is enthusiastic
and the treatment is new, the psychological impact
creates a favorable impression. Any benefit may be attributed to the new therapy rather than the state of
mind which is really responsible.

Vasomotor rhinitis is the name given to the blockage
of one or the other nostril, often alternating, that occurs
particularly on lying down when the mucous membrane becomes congested. It is a very common condition and does not appear to give rise to headache unless
sinusitis takes over, despite reports to the contrary.

TEETH AS A SOURCE OF HEAD PAIN

An infected tooth commonly causes pain locally, and
pain may be referred to the second or third division of
the trigeminal nerve. Thus, an infection of a tooth or a
root fragment remaining in the gum may cause pain in
the entire lower jaw and lower gum or in the cheek,
upper jaw, and upper gum depending on its location.

At the risk of oversimplifying the problem, it could be said that a constant aching pain in the lower jaw is almost always caused by the teeth; in the upper jaw and cheek, sometimes, and in the forehead, never. A routine dental examination may not disclose the trouble, and X rays of the gums and jaws are usually necessary. If the site of the pain is in a tooth or is close to the surface of the gum, the pain will often be made worse by hot and cold substances in the mouth.

Pain in the ear and temple may be caused indirectly by dental problems, often compounded by the problem of jaw clenching in tense or anxious patients. The jaw bone is hinged on each side to permit normal chewing movements. If the fingers are placed in front of the ears and slightly below them, the gliding movement of the jaw bone at this point can be felt with each bite. When the bite is unbalanced by loss of the molars at the back of the gums, on one or both sides, the individual has to chew on one side only, or to use the incisor teeth in the front for chewing. Either way a strain is set up in the jaw joint opposite the side used for chewing. If, in addition, the patient is tense, the habit of clenching the teeth may aggravate that tendency. The joint under constant pressure often becomes painful so that tenderness may be felt in front of the ear and pain may radiate up to the temple or down over the face on the affected side. Sometimes the ear may feel blocked and deaf on that side because the tube running from the ear to the nose (the Eustachian tube), which lies behind the jaw joint, becomes obstructed. If the joint deteriorates, a distinct clicking sensation may be felt or heard over it with each biting movement. This constellation of symptoms is known as Costen's syndrome, and may be corrected by balancing the bite. The treatment is essentially within the province of the dental surgeon, but the problem of nervous tension and jaw-clenching may require additional psychological help and relaxation therapy.

In Costen's syndrome and in jaw-clenchers, the pain may become so severe as to resemble tic douloureux. It is said that some patients with typical tic douloureux may also respond to correction of the bite, but I have not observed any instance of this happening.

NECK HEADACHE

There are at least four ways in which troubles in the neck may cause headache, but, to lay my cards on the table at the outset, I consider that none of them is a very common cause of headache. This defensive attitude is adopted because there are many who believe that almost all headache comes from the neck and can be cured by manipulating the neck, just as there are those who believe that most headaches can be cured by nasal surgery, the treatment of allergies, or psychotherapy. Would that it were so simple. If it were, there would be no need for a book of this sort, no need for the classification and diagnosis of headache, and no need for further research into the many different types of headache. First, the four ways in which neck disturbances *can* cause headache.

The neck consists of seven separate bones (vertebrae) separated by disks which act as shock absorbers (see Figures 1, 2). The bones touch one another at two points where they form joints—first, where vertebral body meets vertebral body (the neurocentral joints) and, second, where the side processes of the vertebrae, which project laterally like wings, connect with one another, resembling the flying buttresses of a cathedral (interpedicular joints). Between the two sets of joints is a gap traversed by the nerves which pass through to join the

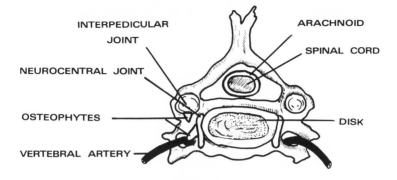

Figure 2. Pressure on nerve roots and the vertebral artery in the neck. A cervical vertebra viewed from above. When a disk between two vertebrae degenerates, bone spurs (osteophytes) project from the interpedicular and neurocentral joints and may compress the nerve root which runs between them as it leaves the spinal canal on its way from the spinal cord to other structures in the neck. The vertebral arteries are also vulnerable as they travel in a canal in the bone and may be narrowed by the pressure of osteophytes as the neck is turned.

spinal cord. Branches of the upper three of these nerves pass over the back of the head (Figure 1), while other branches supply the joints of the neck. If the vertebrae are displaced or if the disks degenerate, an arthritic change may take place in one or both types of joint or the nerve roots may be compressed. When the joints degenerate, they form little spikes of bone termed osteophytes (Figure 2). Some osteophytes extend outward from the neurocentral joints, and others extend inward from the interpedicular joints, so that the gap for the passage of the nerve root becomes smaller and smaller until the root becomes compressed. For any of these reasons, nerve impulses may be set up in these roots which give rise to pain over the upper neck and back of the head. Thus the neck has to be considered as a

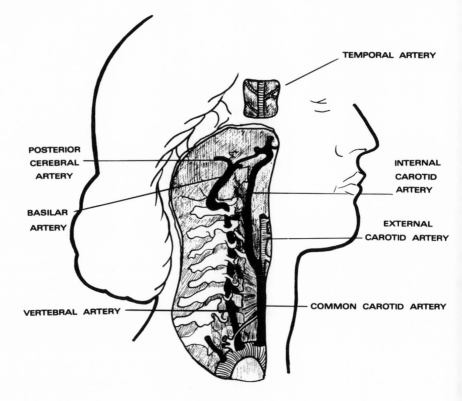

TEMPORAL ARTERY

POSTERIOR CEREBRAL ARTERY

BASILAR ARTERY

VERTEBRAL ARTERY

INTERNAL CAROTID ARTERY

EXTERNAL CAROTID ARTERY

COMMON CAROTID ARTERY

Figure 3. Main arteries of the head. The common carotid artery branches to form the internal carotid artery supplying blood to most of the brain, and the external carotid artery (crosshatched in diagram) which supplies the face and scalp. One of the branches of the external carotid artery commonly affected by migraine is the temporal artery, felt in front of the ear (shown a little larger than life in the diagram). The vertebral arteries run up through canals on each side of the cervical vertebrae and join to form the basilar artery which supplies blood to the brain-stem (and the back part of the brain through the posterior cerebral artery).

cause of any pain extending over the back of the head, particularly if it becomes worse on neck movement. Some conditions, such as whiplash injury to the neck or rheumatoid arthritis, are particularly liable to affect the upper neck and refer pain to the back of the head.

The second form of headache which can arise from the upper part of the neck is a pain shooting to the eye and forehead, related to neck posture. The reason for this is that the nerve fibers which have passed through the bone gap to the spinal cord make connection with nerve cells which also receive nerves from the eye and forehead (Figure 1). Hence, any sudden movement of the neck can cause a pain in the eye and forehead even though the origin is in the upper neck. It must be stressed that there is no known way for disturbance of the lower neck to cause pain to be felt in the head.

A third form of headache which is conceivably of neck origin and remains highly controversial is "cervical migraine." The theory behind this concept is based on the fact that the vertebral arteries pass through canals in the neck bones on their way upward to the skull (Figures 2,3). If the osteophytes described above extend outward sufficiently from the neurocentral joints, they can push the vertebral artery out of its normal path so that it runs a zigzag course as it ascends. If a person with this problem turns his neck sharply, such as a driver looking backward when the car is backing up, the flow in the vertebral arteries may be impaired, a condition called vertebro-basilar insufficiency. This can give rise to a pain in the back of the head together with symptoms coming from the parts of the brain deprived of blood, such as blurring of vision or the sensation of flashing lights in front of the eyes, pins and needles around the mouth and down the body, giddiness, slurred speech, loss of balance, and weakness of the

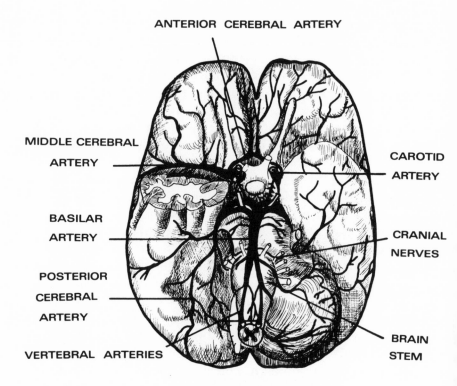

ANTERIOR CEREBRAL ARTERY

MIDDLE CEREBRAL ARTERY

CAROTID ARTERY

BASILAR ARTERY

CRANIAL NERVES

POSTERIOR CEREBRAL ARTERY

VERTEBRAL ARTERIES

BRAIN STEM

Figure 4. Arteries bringing blood to the brain. The brain viewed from below with part of the brain cut away on the left to show the anterior and middle cerebral arteries branching from the internal carotid artery. A part of the hind-brain, the cerebellum, has also been removed on the left side of the diagram to show how the basilar artery divides into the posterior cerebral arteries, supplying blood to the back part of the brain, which is responsible for vision.

legs. The most dramatic example of this I have come across was a man marching past a review point where some dignitary was taking the salute. When the order "eyes right" was given, he turned his head smartly to the right, immediately felt weak in the legs and fell heavily to the ground.

It has been postulated that the same sort of thing may happen in less dramatic form to patients with milder degenerations of the neck disks and joints and produce a form of migraine. The theory behind this is that the network of nerve filaments around the vertebral arteries may be stimulated when the artery is compressed by neck movement, thus setting up a slow-motion version of the above symptoms including headache, called "cervical migraine."

There is no doubt that a form of migraine involves the vertebral arteries and the basilar artery which is formed by their junction (see Figure 4). This is described in a later chapter as "basilar migraine." What is in dispute is whether degenerative changes in the neck can cause migraine. Basilar migraine occurs most commonly in young women who usually have completely normal necks. Vertebro-basilar insufficiency, on the other hand, usually occurs in older patients, who have degenerative changes in the neck but do not suffer from migraine.

There have been many claims that migraine can be cured or relieved by manipulating the neck, but I know of no controlled experiment on this subject. I have certainly seen many patients with migraine and other forms of headache who have not responded to manipulation of the neck. Along with most of my colleagues, I cannot find any real evidence for the concept of "cervical migraine."

The last of the possible "neck headaches" appears to

be more common and understandable. This is a muscle-contraction or tension headache occurring when the patient holds his or her neck stiffly. Many individuals hold their necks rigidly at the best of times, and this tendency is reinforced if they hear a crackling or crunching noise when they move their necks. This sound is caused by osteophytes at the site of disk degeneration and may induce a feeling of apprehension so that the neck muscles contract reflexly to stabilize the neck. If patients view their own X rays, commonly adorned by arrows pointing to the most decrepit areas, without the knowledge that most necks look like that after a few decades of hard wear, the feeling of degeneration is accentuated and the neck is held more rigidly than before. Such muscular contraction causes pain in the back of the head as well as in the neck and may spread to involve other scalp muscles with the development of generalized headache. The management of this problem must include the neck condition as well as the tension state secondary to it.

In short, there are a few headaches which arise from the neck. These may respond to heat, traction of the neck, neck manipulation, the wearing of a collar, or an injection of local anesthetic or cortisone into the offending joints or nerves. Occasionally they may require an operation to remove disks in the neck, to free nerve roots, or even to sever the nerve roots if other measures fail. There are many other forms of headache, the great majority of which bear no other relation to the neck than a certain geographical proximity and respond to manipulation in direct proportion to the personality of the manipulator and the mystique which surrounds his or her performance.

4

A Box of Bone and Its Remarkable Contents

The skull is a box of bone which opens into the spinal canal through a large opening in its base. The bony framework is lined with membranes containing cerebrospinal fluid so that in effect the brain floats in fluid which helps to support it. The membranes and their contained fluid extend down the spinal canal, cushioning the spinal cord from the bone around it. The crystal-clear fluid is made by the filtering of blood through loops of fine vessels *(choroid plexus)* contained in two large cavities, one in each hemisphere of the brain, known as the "lateral ventricles" (Figure 5). The fluid passes from the lateral ventricles into the third ventricle, a slitlike cavity in the center of the brain, and from there flows downward in a canal called the "aqueduct" (in tribute to ancient Roman plumbing) to the fourth ventricle at the back of the brain. From there the fluid spills out holes in the sides and back of the fourth ventricle into cisterns which surround the base of the brain. Some of the fluid then passes into the spinal canal enclosed by a filmy sheath known as the arachnoid to bathe the spinal cord. The greater part of the fluid moves up and over the surface of the brain in the subarachnoid space until it reaches a large vein running from front to back at the top of the brain where the fluid is reabsorbed back into the blood stream (Figure 5). There is thus a continual circulation of fresh fluid through and around the brain. Assuming there is no obstruction to the free flow of fluid, the pressure is determined by the rate of formation and reabsorption

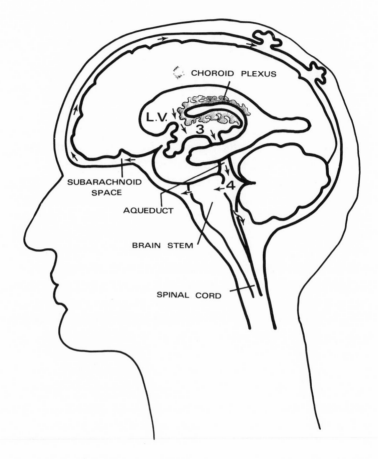

Figure 5. The circulation of cerebrospinal fluid. Cerebrospinal fluid is formed by a network of fine blood vessels (choroid plexus) within the cavities (ventricles) of the brain. The fluid passes from the lateral ventricles (L.V.), one on each side of the brain, into the third ventricle (3). It flows through the aqueduct into the fourth ventricle (4) and then spills out into the subarachnoid space to bathe the brain and spinal cord. The fluid passes over the surface of the brain (arrows) to be absorbed into a large vein at the top of the skull.

of the cerebrospinal fluid. If the flow of fluid is interrupted anywhere along its path, the pressure inside the ventricles increases rapidly, a process known as hydrocephalus. In the infant, before the bones of the skull have joined together, the head may grow larger as the result of hydrocephalus. In the older child and adult whose bones have united, the box of bone becomes rigid and cannot expand. The increasing pressure may, however, give rise to headache.

The blood vessels run upward through the neck to the brain. The carotid arteries are on each side of the neck where their pulsation can be felt (Figure 3). The vertebral arteries are partly contained in a canal of bone within the side wings of the vertebrae (Figures 2, 3). Once inside the skull, the carotid arteries branch to form the cerebral arteries. The two vertebral arteries unite to form the basilar artery which later divides to form the posterior cerebral arteries (Figure 4). The large arteries at the base of the brain are extremely sensitive to pain when they are stretched or dilated. The carotid arteries commonly give rise to pain behind the eyes. The basilar artery and its branches may refer pain to the back of the head.

A number of layers of tissue which wrap around the brain and envelop it are known as the meninges. There is a hard membrane, the dura, lining the inner surface of the skull. Next comes the arachnoid, named for its likeness to the delicacy of a spider's web, which contains the cerebrospinal fluid. Finally, the pia is attached to the brain and constitutes its containing outer surface. Inflammation of the meninges is known as meningitis and may cause severe headache and stiffness of the neck. Irritation of the meninges by blood spilled into the subarachnoid space from a ruptured blood vessel produces an intense headache of sudden onset which resembles that of meningitis. It may come on so quickly that it feels like a blow on the head. A child with a severe infection of any sort, such as tonsillitis, may develop a headache and stiff neck without any inflammation of the meninges. This is caused by overproduction of cerebrospinal fluid and is called meningism. Sometimes it is difficult to be certain on clinical examination whether a child or adult has meningitis, hemorrhage into the subarachnoid space, or simply meningism. For this reason a sample of the fluid may have to be taken from the spinal canal (by a process known as lumbar puncture) to be examined under the microscope and subjected to chemical analysis.

Most remarkable of all the contents of the box of bone is the brain itself. Its convoluted appearance and jelly-like consistency may appear to the casual viewer to be a frail and undignified vessel to contain the mind of man, and yet we live in our brain, and all the other parts of the body are servants to it. The sole purpose of the lungs, heart, and blood vessels is to supply the brain with oxygen and nourishment so that it can think for us. The sole purpose of our bones and joints and muscles is to provide messengers to do the bidding of the brain. The brain contains ten thousand million nerve cells which are interconnected like complex electronic circuitry which would make a computer blanch were it suitably endowed. Regrettably, the brain does share one attribute with modern technology, its built-in obsolescence. It has been estimated that brain nerve cells die at the rate of about ten thousand each day from the age of sixteen onward. However, a rapid calculation will convince the faint-hearted that there are more than enough cells to last a lifetime. Curiously enough, the brain is insensitive to pain, so that diseases affecting it cause headache only when they displace blood vessels or block the flow of fluid, as in the case of brain tumors, or if they irritate the meninges. Inflammation of the brain, encephalitis, is associated with headache because of swelling of the brain or involvement of the meninges in the inflammatory reaction. For this reason infections of the brain by viruses are often called meningo-encephalitis.

LOW PRESSURE HEADACHE

If the pressure of the fluid surrounding and supporting the brain is lowered, the brain no longer "floats" at the same level, and strain is placed on the blood vessels which then have to help in maintaining its position. This strain results in a headache which is worse when sitting or standing, because the brain tends to sag downward when the head is upright. Such a headache may develop after a lumbar puncture. Lumbar puncture is a method of sampling the contents of the cerebrospinal fluid by inserting a fine needle between the vertebrae in the lower part of the back (lumbar region). The area is numbed first by the injection of local anesthetic so that the procedure is not as drastic as it may sound. In skilled hands and with a modest degree of luck, the procedure may end with the patient asking, "When are you going to begin?" just as the needle is being removed.

No matter how skilled the doctor, about ten milliliters of fluid has to be withdrawn for all the appropriate tests. The patient has to make up that amount of fluid afterward and is advised to rest in bed for twenty-four hours. It is best for the first few hours for the patient to be in the prone position (lying on his stomach). In this position the small puncture made in the arachnoid is uppermost, and the normal curve of the spine tends to close off the puncture wound. If the patient lies on his or her back on a soft mattress, the puncture wound may open so that fluid can seep into the tissues. In any event, some patients do develop a headache after lumbar puncture. In this case, the only solution is to keep lying down and drink plenty of fluid until the cerebrospinal fluid is replenished and the brain floats again in its usual buoyant fashion.

HIGH PRESSURE HEADACHE

Any abnormality in the circulation of the cerebrospinal fluid which prevents its flow through the ventricles and canal system of the brain, or a blockage of the great vein which absorbs the fluid, will cause an increase in intracranial pressure. The arteries may be placed under tension and respond by causing a headache which is worse on bending forward or jolting or jarring of the head. This will be discussed in the next chapter which deals with the question which every headache sufferer asks at some time, "Do I have a brain tumor?"

In addition to cerebrospinal fluid outside the brain substance, each cell in the brain contains fluid, and minute quantities of fluid probably lie between the cells. If the fluid content of the cells increases, the whole brain may swell, increasing the pressure within the skull or cranium. This is known as cerebral edema or "water on the brain." A 2.5 percent increase in brain "water" can cause a fourfold increase in intracranial pressure.

WATER ON THE BRAIN

This expression has fallen from common usage, but the naïve phrase expresses the problem succinctly. I remember a joke from childhood of the "I say, I say, I say" variety which ran something like this:

> "There I was at the North Pole, face to face with an enormous bear, and had no gun."
> "What did you do?"
> "I hurled an icicle at his head."
> "Did the icicle kill him?"
> "No, but the bear eventually died of water on the brain!"

I wondered then what exactly was meant by water on the brain. I doubt if I would have appreciated the explanation—that the water was not on the brain but in the brain and was indeed contained in each cell of the brain. There are many factors which may help to retain fluid in brain cells. Perhaps we could start with one related to the bear's environment. High doses of vitamin A can cause swelling of the brain. Vitamin A is concentrated in the livers of fish, seals, and animals such as bears and huskies living in the Arctic or Antarctic. You may recall being given cod-liver oil as a child to increase your body stores of vitamins A and D. Eskimos are well aware of the dangers of eating excessive quantities of liver, but this fact was unknown to some of the early explorers. Four to eight hours after eating a meal of seal liver, the Arctic or Antarctic gourmand may experience severe headache, giddiness, vomiting, and diarrhea, followed after some days by peeling of the skin. Sir John Cleland and Dr. R. V. Southcott recount the case of Mawson and his companion, Mertz, who probably suffered from this condition in the Antarctic expedition of 1911–1914 after they were forced to eat their dogs, including the livers. Mertz subsequently suffered vomiting, diarrhea, and delirium. Both were troubled by "wholesale peeling of skin all over our bodies." Mertz eventually died after a convulsion.

Swelling of the brain may be a feature of lead poisoning and has been reported occasionally after treatment with the antibiotic tetracycline, the urinary antiseptic nalidixic acid, and the long-term use of steroids such as cortisone. Brain swelling resulting from steroids is paradoxical because one of the most rapid ways known to reduce swelling of the brain is to give large doses of cortisonelike substances. Either a deficiency or an excess of cortisone, which is made by the adrenal glands, may be associated with brain swelling. Other hormone changes may also be responsible. One of the most interesting is the rare occurrence in plump young women, pregnant women, or women taking the contraceptive pill. There are many other causes of headache of which this is one of the least common, so there is no need for any woman to leap to the conclusion that she has the most obscure of all the causes. Moreover, when it does occur it responds so well to treatment that the condition is generally known as benign intracranial hypertension.

Brain swelling may appear after head injury or brain surgery or when a large blood vessel to the brain has become blocked. Prompt control of brain swelling by steroids or by the intravenous infusion of mannitol or glycerol, which absorb fluid from the tissues, has been a major factor in improving the recovery rate in all of these serious situations.

BLOOD PRESSURE

Our discussion of pressure has so far covered pressure inside the skull (intracranial pressure), pressure of the fluid surrounding the brain (cerebrospinal fluid pressure), and pressure within the brain tissue itself. All of these are obviously interdependent and in turn are linked with the pressure in the arteries which supply the brain with blood since the arteries provide the only way fluid can enter the cranium.

There is no doubt that a sudden increase in blood pressure to high levels will cause severe headache. In the kidney disease, acute nephritis, the inflamed kidney manufactures a substance which causes the blood pressure to rise sharply. Other forms of high blood pressure may also come on acutely. A small tumor of the adrenal glands (with the glorious name of pheochromocytoma) can release epinephrine and norepinephrine into the blood stream intermittently. When it does, the heart rate increases, which may be felt as "palpitations" in the chest, the hands become shaky, and the blood pressure shoots up. The patient commonly feels a sudden sharp ache in the back of the head or over the top of the head which does not usually last long, probably because the blood vessels of the brain and scalp soon constrict in response to the circulating epinephrine and the patient then looks pale. This type of headache is remarkably similar to that described in Chapter 2 as benign sex headache, occurring at the moment of orgasm, in which case, too, epinephrine may suddenly be released. A third form of headache in which epinephrine causes an upsurge of blood pressure has been observed in patients taking a certain type of drug for depression. The brain's content of epinephrine and norepinephrine, and possibly another substance called serotonin, is low in states of depression. Normally they are broken down in the body by an enzyme, monoamine oxidase (MAO). In order to allow their levels to build up, this enzyme is put out of action by drugs known as MAO inhibitors. These are extremely effec-

tive in improving the patient's mood, but if any substance like epinephrine enters the body or is manufactured in excess inside the body, it cannot be destroyed
before it causes an acute rise of blood pressure. Cheese
and some kinds of red wine contain chemicals which
are either precursors of epinephrine or release it in the
body, and these substances are therefore forbidden to
any patient taking MAO inhibitors. Before this was
recognized, there were reports of patients attending
cheese and wine tasting parties who suffered a devastating headache as a result. Any person taking these
pills must be extremely careful about taking any other
form of medication at the same time. Even the inhalation of a spray to clear the nose may be hazardous
because some nasal sprays contain substances allied to
epinephrine.

Apart from these acute episodes, the relationship between headache and high blood pressure is probably
indirect. It is said that people with high blood pressure
are likely to awaken with a headache in the morning,
but it passes off as they get up and about. Certainly,
migraine attacks increase in frequency in patients
whose blood pressure rises, and control of the blood
pressure subsequently improves the headaches. It is
uncertain whether a modest increase in blood pressure
will actually induce headaches in an individual who has
previously been free from headache. Only about one-
half of patients with high blood pressure complain of
headache, and their pressure readings are no higher
than those that are headache-free. It is probable that
the knowledge that blood pressure is higher than it
should be is sufficient cause to induce a tension headache in some people, and that the caliber of the vessels
fluctuates more widely as blood pressure increases,
making the individual more susceptible to vascular

headaches. Adequate control of blood pressure can therefore be regarded as an important point in the management of headache.

BIG STROKES AND LITTLE STROKES

A stroke is a "stroke of fate" that leaves someone disabled in some way as a result of sudden damage to the nervous system. In practice the term is usually applied to a blockage of a blood vessel or a hemorrhage into part of the brain which leaves a patient paralyzed down one side. If the right side of the body becomes weak in a right-handed person, the power of speech may also be impaired since the connections between the brain and the body are crossed and the left hemisphere of the brain is responsible not only for movement of the right side of the body but also for the planning and execution of the complex intellectual skills of speech, writing, and calculation. The most common single factor underlying the tendency to have a stroke is sustained untreated high blood pressure, although other factors, such as the level of fatty substances in the blood and hereditary susceptibility, also play an important role.

It is not difficult to see how a hemorrhage into part of the brain can cause headache, simply by occupying space in one hemisphere, thus displacing pain-sensitive blood vessels. If blood should be spilt into the ventricular system so that it becomes mixed with the cerebrospinal fluid, it will pass down the spinal canal in the subarachnoid space, irritating the meninges, and causing neck pain and stiffness as well as headache. After some days, the blood may gravitate to the lowest part of the spinal canal. It then causes pain in the back and legs by producing a sterile inflammation of the nerve roots. This is called subarachnoid hemorrhage because of the plane into which the bleeding occurs, in which the blood cells mingle with the cerebrospinal fluid. It may complicate any cerebral hemorrhage but is most commonly caused by bleeding from an aneurysm, a "blow-out" on an artery. An aneurysm looks like a small balloon, the size of a cherry or even a red currant. Some people are born with these little sacs on the arteries, or at least with a predisposing weakness of the vessel wall, which may accompany them throughout life without causing a moment's trouble. In others, particularly those who develop high blood pressure, the aneurysm may enlarge and eventually rupture, often at a time of strenuous physical exertion. Since the bleeding takes place in a high-pressure system, it is potentially dangerous and requires careful assessment by a neurological unit. A subarachnoid hemorrhage can also arise from a low-pressure system (from abnormal cerebral veins) if the patient happens to be born with a cerebral angioma or arterio-venous malformation. An angioma is a collection of blood vessels in which blood passes through large channels from arteries to veins. It looks like a cluster of varicose veins overlying the surface of the brain. If the doctor listens with his stethoscope over the skull or over the eye he can sometimes hear a murmuring sound as blood is shunted through large blood vessels in the angioma. The condition may be present throughout life without any complications and, if it does bleed, the hazards are much less than that of an aneurysm because of the low pressure in the system. There has been much written in the medical literature about angiomas underlying migraine-type headache. This does not appear to be a valid relationship because only 5 percent of patients with proven angiomas have suffered from migraine headache, and this proportion is no greater than that of the general population.

A more common cause of stroke is a thrombosis, or clot, in a vessel narrowed by the accumulation of a fatty deposit called atheroma. Long before any stroke occurs there may be warning symptoms of transient weakness in one side of the body, of pins and needles, blurring of vision, giddiness, loss of balance, and a host of other temporary disabilities. These symptoms may indicate insufficiency of blood flow in the cerebral vessels. They are brought into the present discussion simply because they can be accompanied by headache. The ache is in the back of the head, if the vertebral and basilar arteries are momentarily obstructed, or on one side of the head, if flow is suddenly diminished in one carotid artery. The occurrence of odd neurological symptoms in association with headache, particularly a one-sided headache, may suggest the diagnosis of migraine and may require all the skill of the neurologist to make the correct diagnosis in doubtful cases. The cause of headache in vascular insufficiency is probably dilatation of extra blood channels which open up to bypass the blocked artery and convey blood to the brain through a roundabout route. Vascular insufficiency is treated by opening up the narrowed arteries if the obstruction is in a place accessible to surgery or by preventing the clumping together of small particles in blood known as platelets, if no surgical measures are possible, to minimize the possibility of a clot forming in the narrowed artery. It appears that an aspirin tablet taken two or three times daily is as effective as any treatment to stop blood platelets sticking together, and this is now being used as part of the treatment.

Many patients with headache fear that they are more liable to have a stroke than their next door neighbors. This is a groundless fear. Headaches from vascular insufficiency are very uncommon and are associated with

other symptoms. Headaches from other causes are le-
gion.

BLOOD VESSELS AS A TARGET

Much has been said so far about blood vessels. They are
pain-sensitive, they may dilate to give rise to headache,
and they are very vulnerable to any changes in the
blood they contain. Any reduction of oxygen in the
blood stream makes the vessels dilate, which thus increases the blood flow and makes more oxygen available to the tissues. Any accumulation of carbon dioxide
has a similar effect but is rather more potent in dilating
the vessels. After a convulsion or epileptic fit, in which
breathing stops momentarily, the oxygen supply to the
brain is reduced for some seconds and the carbon dioxide level of the blood increases. The vessels therefore
dilate and the patient awakens with a headache. In a
less dramatic situation, the same mechanism may apply. A crowded meeting in a relatively small room on
a winter's night with all the windows closed—a perfect
setting for the respiratory seesaw to swing—the oxygen
goes down, the carbon dioxide goes up. The vessels
dilate and the headache starts. The fact that so many
headaches are present on waking in the morning may
also be related to the fact that the carbon dioxide content of the blood slowly increases during sleep causing
vessels to dilate. "His face was flushed with sleep." It
may soon grow pale with headache.

Any poison which prevents the normal delivery of
oxygen to the tissues will have the same effect. Carbon
monoxide is the commonest example.

In 1931, Charles Kingsford Smith set off to fly from
Australia to England in an Avro Avian named Southern
Cross Minor in an attempt to break the previous record

time for the flight. As he was approaching Rangoon he twice wrote in his logbook that he was suffering from acute headaches and had suffered a spell of dizziness. After leaving Rangoon, he was halfway across the Bay of Bengal when he wrote, "I feel awful! Think I've got a touch of sunstroke." By the time he had reached Calcutta he felt very weak and sick. On arrival at Karachi, he was unable to sleep and recorded that he had "a rotten night . . . my head bashed away like a bloody drum." His illness became worse as the flight progressed until finally he made an emergency landing in Turkey after writing, "I feel as though I might die before this flight is over . . . must find a place to land . . . if I don't I'll crash for sure." After recovering he flew on to Athens, with a recurrence of his symptoms on the way. It was in Athens that the leak in the exhaust pipe was discovered, a leak that had allowed carbon monoxide to diffuse into the cockpit and incapacitate him with headaches and dizzy spells.

Under normal circumstances the brain obtains its energy only from glucose. Severe lowering of blood sugar levels means that the brain cannot obtain nourishment and the resulting symptoms are similar to those of shortage of oxygen. This occurs most commonly in diabetic patients who give themselves more insulin than is necessary for their present diet or take an excessive number of pills to lower the blood sugar. Curiously enough, low blood sugar may follow an excessive intake of sugar or other carbohydrates. This is called carbohydrate intolerance. After a high carbohydrate meal the blood sugar may rise rapidly but may fall after an hour or two to subnormal levels and cause confusion, trembling, unpleasant abdominal sensations, and headache. The same sequence may be found in patients who have had part of their stomach removed for peptic ulcers.

Vascular headaches, particularly migraine, may be triggered by low blood sugar.

The blood vessels are also a target for any toxins circulating in the body. With most severe infections, a vascular headache contributes to the patient's misery. When there is a reaction to injections of typhoid vaccine or a smallpox vaccination, a throbbing headache is a common accompaniment. The common hangover headache is a toxic dilatation of intracranial vessels, caused by the breakdown products of alcohol.

One interesting cause of headache is the rebound dilatation of vessels which follow the use of any substance which causes them to constrict. Any agent which narrows vessels is called a vasoconstrictor, the commonest being caffeine. Caffeine is a component of headache powders or pills known as A.P.C., standing for aspirin, phenacetin (or paracetamol), and caffeine. Some people take these as a pick-me-up because of their caffeine content. Caffeine is a stimulant as well as a constrictor of blood vessels. As the effect wears off, the user feels let down. The cerebral vessels then dilate again so that a dull headache appears and the stage is then set for taking a few more A.P.C. pills. This is a common vicious circle of caffeine-intake and caffeine-withdrawal headache. The same cycle may trouble habitual coffee and tea drinkers who experience withdrawal symptoms including headache if more than a few hours elapse between coffee and tea breaks. The habitual taking of analgesic tablets, whether or not they contain caffeine, is potentially dangerous because their use over a number of years can cause permanent damage to the kidneys.

Some medications are given deliberately to cause dilatation of arteries and so may evoke headache as a side effect. Amyl nitrite or nitroglycerin (glyceryl trinitrate) is given to patients whose coronary arteries are narrowed sufficiently to cause pain or tightness in the chest on exertion (angina pectoris). The pills are effective in easing the discomfort in the chest but may cause a throbbing headache. Workers who come into contact with nitroglycerin or other nitrates or with other vasodilator substances may complain of headache. Histamine dilates vessels and has been used experimentally to cause a headache so the effect could be studied. It is possible that histamine release in allergic reactions may sometimes account for headache. Certain drugs give headache as a side effect, particularly those which dilate vessels such as dipyridamole. Of patients who are being treated regularly with indomethacin, an agent which is most effective for the relief of some forms of arthritis and other joint and muscle pains, 25 to 50 percent notice a continual dull headache.

MENINGITIS AND ENCEPHALITIS

Arteries dilate as a part of any inflammatory process, such as an infection of any part of the body. The blood supply to the affected area is thus increased, allowing the white cells of the blood to flock to the area to aid in the body's defenses. Those white cells which die in the struggle with the invaders accumulate as pus. Any inflamed area becomes tense because the dilated vessels leak fluid into the tissues at the site of battle between the infecting organism and body cells. The vessels are thus dilated and displaced by tissue swelling so that they are very sensitive to pressure or to jolting and jarring.

Meningitis is an inflammation of the membranes of the brain, usually caused by bacteria, and starts as a severe headache with neck stiffness, fever, and usually dislike of light (photophobia). The diagnosis may be confirmed by sampling the cerebrospinal fluid by lumbar puncture and the appropriate antibiotic given. The infection gains access to the nervous system through the blood stream but may also invade directly from the ear, nose, or sinuses. Hippocrates in the fifth century B.C. warned that an association of fever with acute pain in the ear was to be dreaded "for there is danger that the man may become delirious and die."

Encephalitis is an infection of the brain itself. It may be an extension of meningitis or may be a viral infection which attacks the brain cells directly. The symptoms are much the same as meningitis, but the patient becomes mentally confused and drowsy earlier in the disease.

There is a much milder form of viral infection, which is also more common, usually called viral meningo-encephalitis because the membranes of the brain and the brain tissue are both involved, or aseptic meningitis because no bacteria can be grown from the fluid. Most severe viral infections cause some degree of meningo-encephalitis. Most children and adults experience headaches with measles, mumps, and influenza, and when the cerebrospinal fluid has been examined at this time, an increase in the number of cells in the fluid indicates that the virus is active in the nervous system. Most of these viral illnesses subside without any complications and many require no treatment other than bed rest and analgesics to relieve headache. The number of serious cases of encephalitis is fortunately small. The persistence of any headache with a fever is nevertheless a reason to call the doctor to see whether further diagnostic tests or active treatment is necessary.

HEADACHE AMONG OLDER PEOPLE

There is a particular form of headache which usually affects patients over the age of fifty-five which is caused by a curious inflammation of blood vessels in the scalp and often in the cerebral vessels as well. The condition is known as temporal arteritis or giant-cell arteritis. It is worth a special mention because it is so uncommon that it may not be thought of until the condition is well advanced, and early treatment is essential in preventing complications which may be serious enough to progress to blindness.

Temporal arteritis is a low-grade inflammation of arteries which usually affects the scalp vessels first, particularly the arteries in the temple; hence, its name. The walls of the arteries become thickened and packed with inflammatory cells including giant cells containing many nuclei which give rise to the alternative name, giant-cell arteritis. It may be accompanied by redness, swelling, and tenderness of the arteries in the scalp, in which case there is little difficulty in diagnosis. The more difficult diagnostic problems are those where the symptoms are simply a dull persistent ache on one or both sides of the head. To complicate the issue, arteries in other parts of the body may be involved, in which case the first symptoms may be a general sensation of being unwell, together with aches and pains in the muscles and joints, like a low-grade influenza. This condition has been called polymyalgia rheumatica, meaning rheumatic aches in the joints and muscles. One rather distinctive symptom of temporal arteritis is aching of the jaw muscles when chewing. This is caused by reduction of the blood supply to these muscles as the arteries become narrowed.

The development of these symptoms or of headache

in this age group warrants a blood count and estimation
of the sedimentation rate of the blood. Blood cells sedi-
ment or separate out under the influence of gravity if
blood is left standing in a test tube with a substance to
prevent it from clotting. This separation can be seen
quite easily as a band of clear plasma above the dense
red color of the packed cells. Normally the cells sedi-
ment at less than twenty millimeters each hour, but in
inflammatory conditions like temporal arteritis the rate
is usually more than forty millimeters each hour, and
may be as fast as one hundred millimeters in one hour.
It is a simple test which can help to confirm the suspicion of temporal arteritis. To make completely certain
of the diagnosis, it is usually necessary to remove a small
section of an affected scalp artery and examine it under
a microscope.

It is most important to diagnose the condition early
because it may spread to intracranial arteries. Unfortunately, it has a predilection for picking out the ophthalmic artery which supplies the retina of the eye. If this
artery is affected, it may clot and vision may be lost in
that eye. This may happen with appalling suddenness.
A wise old dairy farmer was sent to see me after having
lost his eyesight in the right eye only a few days after
developing a headache in the right temple. He had
virtually made his own diagnosis. He said to me, "You
know, it's a funny thing, but the pulse in my right temple just disappeared at the same time as I went blind in
the right eye." This tragedy can often be avoided by
starting treatment with steroids as soon as the diagnosis
is made. It may be necessary to continue treatment for
twelve months or more to hold the condition at bay
while it burns itself out.

We have dealt with a large number of problems,
some minor and some major, which can affect the

magic contents of the white box of bone to produce headaches. Others will be considered in the next chapter on brain tumors and other lumps or bumps which may occupy space in that unyielding box where space is at a premium. Fortunately, nasty causes of headache are rare, but we must never relax our vigilance so that we can spot them before they have time to do any harm.

5
Do I Have a Brain Tumor?

HOW COMMON IS BRAIN TUMOR AS A CAUSE OF HEADACHE?

Not all patients with brain tumors complain of headaches, and certainly only a very small proportion of those with headaches turn out to have tumors. When a headache clinic was established in our hospital in the 1960s we made a careful survey of the diagnoses in the first one thousand patients who had suffered from chronic headaches—that is, a headache problem of long duration. Of these, only one was found to have a cerebral tumor. The figures make it clear that any patient who has suffered from headaches for five, ten, or fifteen years is extremely unlikely to have a brain tumor and that, if he or she does, it may well be a coincidental finding not related to the complaint of headache.

Brain tumors are really quite uncommon. They constitute about one-fifth of all tumors in childhood, but in this age group tumors of any sort are fortunately rare anyway. In adults, only 1 percent of all tumors are found in the brain. What are the chances of an individual developing a brain tumor? To take the highest possible incidence first, about 2 percent of all routine postmortem examinations show a brain tumor to have been present during life. Many of these are small and have not given rise to any symptoms during life. Others are secondary deposits which have arisen from some other part of the body and have not grown primarily in the brain. In a sample population, the chances of anyone

72

having any sort of tumor affecting the brain or spinal cord are about one in two thousand.

The important task for the doctor is to identify the pattern of headache and the associated symptoms which give rise to the suspicion of a tumor. Patients with these symptoms may be given special tests, which will be described later. Those who have a pattern of headache completely different from that associated with brain tumors may not require any investigation at all. Whether the possibility of tumor is excluded on clinical grounds or by the results of special tests, it is important that the patient be completely reassured because fear of a brain tumor is a very real thing for most patients with headache.

TYPES OF BRAIN TUMOR

Tumors may be benign or malignant, primary or secondary, operable or inoperable. A tumor is a collection of body cells which multiply indiscriminately without the control or organization which characterizes normal growth. A tumor is said to be benign if it grows slowly, pushing other tissues aside, and confines its development to a single site. If the tumor grows rapidly and invades and destroys normal tissues, it is said to be malignant. Fragments of malignant tumors may separate and travel elsewhere in the body by way of the lymph ducts or the blood stream to set up colonies of abnormal cells which are known as secondary tumors. The malignant process in general is called cancer.

Many benign tumors of the brain can be completely removed with excellent results by a neurosurgeon. Examples of these are tumors arising from the meninges, called meningiomas (accounting for some 20 percent of all brain tumors), tumors of the pituitary gland (about

8 percent of the total), cysts above the pituitary gland (3 percent), and fibrous growths growing from the eighth cranial nerve, the nerve of hearing (8 percent). Some tumors that have all the characteristics of a benign tumor nevertheless lie deeply within the brain or infiltrate between normal structures so that their complete removal would result in severe damage to the brain. They may therefore be inoperable although classified as benign. Most of these tumors grow from the glial (connective tissue) cells of the brain, which perform a supporting function for the nerve cells, and are therefore called gliomas. Glial cell tumors range (in microscopic appearance) from benign to highly malignant. They account for about 45 percent of all brain tumors. About 8 percent of brain tumors turn out to be secondary deposits from cancer elsewhere in the body, particularly from the lung (which is responsible for 65 percent), breast, gastrointestinal tract, and kidney.

The task of the neurologist and neurosurgeon is first to determine whether or not a brain tumor is present, then, if a tumor is found, to localize it carefully and to determine its nature to ascertain whether or not it can be completely or partially removed without avoidable damage to normal tissues. It is desirable to make the diagnosis as soon as possible, although in most cases it is true to say that a tumor which can be successfully removed today could be equally successfully removed in a few months' time. This may not hold true if the growth of the tumor has imperiled vital structures, which can make operating a matter of urgency. Some tumors in particular must be diagnosed early to obtain the best results. One such example is an eighth nerve tumor, which causes loss of hearing in one ear years before it produces headache. It should be diagnosed when investigating the deafness and not left to wait for headache or other symptoms. Other brain tumors do have headaches as a main symptom.

A SINISTER PATTERN OF HEADACHE

A brain tumor does not cause headache until it pushes arteries aside, thus placing them under tension, or until it increases intracranial pressure by other means. In some parts of the brain a tumor may grow to a considerable size without doing either of these things. If, on the other hand, the tumor lies in or around the ventricles or aqueduct through which the cerebrospinal fluid flows (see Figure 5), it causes distension of the ventricles. The blood vessels around the ventricles are displaced and headache appears as an early symptom. Headache is a feature sooner or later in 90 percent of brain tumors. The pain may be felt in the front or back of the head or in the whole head. It is usually intermittent and does not often approach the intensity of severe migraine or meningitis or subarachnoid hemorrhage, described in the previous chapter. The ache is commonly made worse by coughing, sneezing, or straining, but this may also be a feature of any intracranial vascular headache, including hangover headache. The most distinctive feature of this headache pattern is that it arises in a person not previously subject to headaches or one who experiences a complete change in the pattern of any pre-existing headache. The headache also progressively becomes worse. If, in addition, the patient yawns or becomes drowsy at inappropriate times, or develops any symptoms of neurological damage, the suspicion of a tumor greatly increases.

Almost always, some form of neurological deficit accompanies the growth of a brain tumor. Some deficits may be obvious, such as a progressive weakness or numbness of one side of the body, impairment of vision, difficulty in speaking, or loss of balance. More subtle may be loss of the sense of smell, the gradual onset of deafness in one ear, impairment of mental faculties, or bursts of irrational behavior. One patient of mine, a young man whose demeanor had previously been impeccable, was visiting Singapore when he startled his friends, as well as the hotel management, by dropping "water bombs" from his hotel room onto guests relaxing on the lawn below. He followed this by throwing empty bottles down an elevator shaft. Such episodes led to his premature return to Sydney where he was found to have a tumor of the frontal lobes of the brain. Any sudden drastic alteration of behavior should lead to suspicion of a brain tumor, although there are, of course, many other possible explanations. The association between any of the above symptoms and headache is not in itself significant, because other disorders such as migraine can be responsible for many perturbing alterations of brain function preceding or accompanying headache. The significant aspect of the brain tumor story is the steady worsening of the headache and neurological impairment. The occurrence of epileptic fits and headache together is a combination that also warrants a thorough investigation.

SOME SPECIAL INVESTIGATIONS

Must I be a guinea pig?
After the most painstaking examination, it is still not possible to be dogmatic about the presence or absence of a brain tumor. If there is an obvious abnormality found on examination, the likelihood may be very high. Swelling of the optic nerve head (papilledema) may be

seen on looking at the interior of the eye with an oph-thalmoscope. This indicates that the ophthalmic veins are not able to drain the fluid away from the retina, a sign of increased intracranial pressure. In itself it does not give any clue as to why the pressure is increased. Other signs may enable a neurologist to point precisely to the site of the disturbance. He may know *where* it is but cannot be certain *what* it is. To confirm the location of the abnormality, to assess its size, to see how it is affecting neighboring structures, and to make steps toward determining its nature, special investigations have to be made. After all, even detectives have to take fingerprints.

The reaction of patients to the suggestion of further tests depends upon their level of knowledge and sophistication as well as their degree of confidence in their doctor. Most people understand why the tests are being made and are glad that the possibility of a tumor is being ruled out if any suspicion has arisen, or that any abnormality is being carefully studied if one has been found. A few adopt a querulous, argumentative, or plaintive attitude, with variations on the theme of "Must I be a guinea pig?" There is no question of any person undergoing these tests as a guinea pig. Any neurological or neurosurgical team of even modest size conducts these tests regularly with a precision that makes them little more adventurous than taking a ride in a train, and in most cases less hazardous than driving one's car to the hospital. The first series of tests described can be done on an outpatient basis and carries no risk whatever. Specialized X rays of the arteries to the brain and of the brain itself are virtually free of risk to anyone who does not have pre-existing disease. If there is disease of the arteries or brain, any risk is minimized by conducting the tests in a logical and orderly sequence. Such a risk is small indeed, compared with the benefit of knowing precisely where the trouble lies and what must be done about it.

The electroencephalogram (EEG)

The EEG or "brain-wave test" is no more disturbing to most people than having their hair set. Having witnessed but never experienced the beauty-parlor routine of rollers and hair dryers, I personally would prefer having an EEG! Electrodes are placed on the head with a little paste, to ensure that they make good contact with the scalp. Activity of brain cells is associated with electrical changes. When groups of cells become synchronized in their activity, the electrical waves are large enough to be recorded from the scalp. The resulting "brain waves" are amplified and then recorded automatically by pens on a moving chart. There is no way that electricity can jump back from the machine to shock the patient.

Normally a rhythm of electrical waves of about ten waves a second, called alpha rhythm, is recorded symmetrically from the back half of the head overlying the part of the brain concerned with sight (the visual cortex). If the eyes are closed, the cells all beat together, like an engine idling in neutral, and the alpha rhythm is picked up. When the eyes are open, each cell has its own task to do and so the group activity is less conspicuous. The patient is therefore asked to open and close his or her eyes at intervals throughout the recording, and the alpha rhythm is seen to wax and wane as a result. An abnormality may show up in the record as an asymmetry in the alpha rhythm or as slower rhythms which are classified as theta and delta. These may be localized to a particular electrode, indicating a disturbance in that region of the brain.

After the routine recording is completed, the patient is asked to breathe fast and deeply for two or three minutes. This washes carbon dioxide out of the lungs and lowers the level circulating in the blood throughout the brain. The blood level of carbon dioxide regulates the caliber of cerebral blood vessels. If the level goes up, the circumference of the arteries increases so that more blood can flow through them. This is called a vasodilator effect. If the level drops, the circumference decreases so that less blood can pass through (vasoconstrictor effect). Overbreathing lowers the carbon dioxide content in the blood which in turn reduces the blood flow through the brain. This is why we may feel faint and dizzy after breathing too much. Any abnormality in the brain waves becomes more obvious when the blood flow slows down.

Near the end of the EEG recording, light may be flashed in the eyes to alter the brain rhythm. The effect of this stroboscopic light is not unpleasant to most people, who are usually intrigued by the colored patterns they see while the light is flashing. The reason for this is that the cells of the visual cortex respond together to each flash of light and beat in unison. The faster the light flashes, the faster the brain cells respond, causing us to "see" a changing spectrum of colors.

Before the days of isotope scanning and the most recent technique of computerized X-ray scanning, which will be described shortly, the EEG was the most useful screening test for a brain tumor. It still gives considerable information and is complementary to the other tests. The procedure takes thirty to sixty minutes to complete. The recording time varies in each laboratory.

Plain X rays

The chest is usually X-rayed at the same time as the skull because a primary cancer of the lung can be responsible for secondary tumors in the brain, and other diseases, like tuberculosis, may also affect both sites. The information obtained from an X ray of the skull is limited. Routine X rays simply show the bones. Any part of the brain which contains calcium also stands out clearly in the X ray. Most tumors do not alter the appearance of bone and therefore do not show up in a plain X ray. The pineal gland, a vestigial structure in the center of the brain, often becomes calcified. It then becomes clearly visible on the skull X ray and indicates whether the midline of the brain is still lying in its normal position or whether it has been pushed out of place by a tumor. Some tumors may absorb calcium, particularly if they are growing slowly. In this case, their position can be seen clearly in plain films of the skull, and some deductions can be made about the type of tumor from the pattern of the calcification.

Ultrasound

If the pineal gland is not calcified, the position in the skull of the midline structures of the brain can be judged from the echo set up by an ultrasonic transmitter. The device is applied to one side of the head, and a recording is made of the waves reflected from more solid areas of the brain and from the skull vault. The technique gives limited information compared with other techniques now available.

Computerized X-ray scanning

The coming of age of the computer provided a means of obtaining much more information from an X-ray beam than was formerly possible. A conventional X ray cannot give a three-dimensional picture because both sides of the skull and all the structures between them are traversed by the X-ray beam. A more precise method of radiography, known as tomography, enables an X-ray beam to focus on a particular plane of the skull but cannot display changes in the brain substance.

The EMI Research Laboratories in England have recently devised a way of overcoming this problem. The invention, computerized transverse axial tomography, relies on a narrow beam of X rays which traverses the skull in a series of steps over a period of five minutes. Two accurately aligned detector units follow the X-ray beam across the head, sensing the transmitted X rays. A reading for each position is recorded, calculated by the computer and printed out or displayed as a picture. In this way small percentage variations of the X-ray penetration can be perceived, which enables the shadows of the ventricles to be seen and the densities of the gray and white matter of the brain to be distinguished. By this method the position and size of a brain tumor can be discovered without risk to the patient, with little more time being spent than with conventional methods, using a comparable amount of radiation. The first machine was installed in 1971, and machines are now in regular use in other hospitals on both sides of the Atlantic. The technique is being further developed, and it is now possible to show cross sections of the body in color on a new American scanner. The only drawback at the moment appears to be the cost of the equipment, but this expenditure may well be justified by reducing the need for other tests.

Isotope scanning
Over the last fifteen years brain scanning by means of radioactive isotopes has overshadowed the EEG in

the diagnosis of brain tumor, but it remains to be seen whether it in turn will be eclipsed by computerized X-ray scanning. It will almost certainly remain the chosen method of screening possible cases of brain tumor and for preliminary localization. A radioactive substance with a short half-life (commonly Technetium 99m,) is injected into a vein and is followed by an array of detectors as it passes up through the neck arteries into the brain. A series of photographs is taken by a special camera to check that the isotope is moving normally through all arteries. This is called dynamic scanning because it shows the circulation in action. Once in the brain, the isotope is taken up by the tissues. It accumulates in large amounts in areas where there are many small blood vessels (such as brain tumors) and leaks into the tissues there. The distribution of the isotope is then determined by a detector moving over the skull which records the amount of radiation given off from each position. The isotope has then left the circulation and remains static in the brain tissues (static scanning). It is thus possible to determine the pattern of blood flow by dynamic scanning, while static scanning detects the presence of any abnormality of blood vessels and tissues. Static scanning detects some 85 percent of all brain tumors. The whole procedure takes about one and one-half hours from the injection into the arm vein to the development of the final pictures. The total body dose of radiation is about the same as that directed at the skull when four standard X-ray views are taken. It is best to avoid isotope scanning in pregnancy.

Arteriography

In order to see the precise position of arteries supplying the brain and to pick up any abnormality in them or in the areas they supply, it is necessary to inject a substance into the blood stream which provides enough contrast on the X rays for the arteries and veins to be seen clearly against the background of the surrounding skull bones. This procedure is called arteriography or angiography. It is used to detect narrowing of blood vessels (by fat deposits, atheroma), local dilatations on blood vessels (aneurysms), or a congenital abnormality of blood vessels (angioma). It also points up any displacement of blood vessels from their normal position and may show a network of fine blood vessels within a tumor. The injected dye may linger within an abnormal area to show up as a "blush" after the remainder of the dye has passed through into the draining veins, thus showing up the tumor.

This method is now widely used for the detection and localization of brain tumors but will probably be employed less for this purpose when computerized X-ray scanning becomes more readily available. It requires hospitalization since the dye is injected into an artery, commonly through a thin plastic tube (catheter) inserted into a groin artery, although a direct injection may be made into the neck arteries. The procedure may be done under a local or, occasionally, general anesthetic. The patient is usually kept in bed for twenty-four hours afterward to ensure that there is no complication at the site of injection. The dye contains iodine and therefore has to be used with caution in anyone allergic to iodine. Arteriography carries little risk for patients with healthy arteries but may precipitate clotting of a cerebral artery or of the artery into which the injection is made in older patients with degeneration of the blood vessels. The complication rate may rise to about 3 percent in this group of patients with known vascular disease.

Air encephalography

The fluid-containing channels within the brain—the ventricles, aqueduct, and cisterns—cannot be seen with conventional radiographic methods but stand out clearly when outlined by air. For this purpose air can be inserted into the fluid to gain information about the size, position, and shape of the ventricles or to see whether there is any obstruction to the free flow of fluid. If previous investigations have not given any indication of a space-occupying mass within the skull and intracranial pressure is not raised, the procedure is done under sedation and a local anesthetic with the patient sitting in a specially designed chair. A lumbar puncture is then done: some five milliliters of air are inserted into the spinal canal and the same amount of cerebrospinal fluid withdrawn. The air bubbles upward in the subarachnoid space around the spinal cord and enters the cisterns and ventricular system within the skull (see Figure 5). An X-ray film is then taken to ensure that the first part of the system is being outlined clearly with air. The procedure of inserting air and then withdrawing fluid is repeated until thirty to thirty-five milliliters of air have entered the spinal canal. The chair is then tilted backward on hinges to form a bed so further films can be taken with the patient in a lying position. After the completion of the air encephalogram, the patient is kept in bed for at least twenty-four hours. Most patients experience headache as soon as they raise their head from the pillow. The cause of this headache is the low pressure of the cerebrospinal fluid. The fluid has to be replenished before the patient can sit up with comfort. Therefore, it is advisable for the patient to keep lying down until all traces of headache have disappeared.

If intracranial pressure is increased because of a tumor or other abnormality, a neurosurgeon can make a small hole in the skull under anesthesia and place a fine needle into one ventricle. This serves the dual purpose of reducing the intracranial pressure and of injecting air directly into the ventricles in a safe manner. The process is known as ventriculography. A liquid which shows up on X rays and is heavier than the cerebrospinal fluid can also be injected if the site of obstruction to the fluid-conducting pathways is still in doubt. This substance will sink down through the fluid and outline the area of obstruction.

WHAT IF I DO HAVE A BRAIN TUMOR?

This section will apply to very few. Most patterns of headache are clearly recognizable as migraine or tension states. If your headache problems have come on recently, are increasing in frequency and severity, and are made worse by coughing or sudden head movement, then you should certainly seek attention from your doctor who will refer you to a neurologist if necessary. After a careful examination, it is quite possible that X rays, an electroencephalogram, and brain scan may be suggested. Should all these tests turn out to be negative, the cause of your headache is unlikely to be a tumor, but some 10 to 20 percent of cerebral tumors may not be detected by this preliminary screening, so that further specialized X-ray investigations may be recommended and hospital admission arranged.

If a tumor is found and localized by these tests, you must then be guided by the neurologist or neurosurgeon who is looking after you. Many types of tumors are benign and may be removed completely with no complications afterward. These include meningiomas, pituitary tumors, and some cystic tumors. An eighth nerve tumor also may be removed easily with very little risk if diagnosed early, but the dangers of the operation increase with the size of the tumor and, if the tumor is large enough to compress the vital parts of the brain which maintain respiration, heart rate, and blood pressure, operation becomes hazardous. Some gliomas, such as the cystic gliomas which are found in the cerebellum in the rear compartment of the skull, may be cured completely by operating. These are a particularly common form of brain tumor in children. Other gliomas may advance rapidly and be quite inoperable. In between these extremes there are many which can be partly removed. Radiotherapy may then be used afterward to retard the growth or destroy remaining tumor cells. Such therapy minimizes or delays a possible recurrence.

About 8 percent of brain tumors are secondary deposits from cancer elsewhere in the body. If there is a single secondary deposit in a position in the brain accessible to the neurosurgeon it may warrant removal, although the odds are that there will be other secondary deposits elsewhere in the body. We all know of some patients who have not had any recurrence after an operation on a secondary tumor. There is an unexplained immune process which sometimes steps in to produce a "miracle cure" in some patients with cancer, unfortunately not very often but frequently enough to give research workers hope that this process might eventually be simulated by treatment in all cases.

6
Headache after Head Injury

The faster and farther man travels, the more likely he is to injure his head. Increasing industrialization adds its share of blows on the head, mitigated to some extent by the use of safety helmets. Head injury may result in a temporary loss of consciousness (concussion), compression of the brain by an enlarging blood clot, or destruction of part of the brain by direct violence. A fracture of the skull by itself may not cause any damage to the brain. If bone fragments are forced inwards, they may press on the brain surface; or, if the line of fracture runs across a large blood vessel in the skull bones, tearing it, the brain may be compressed by hemorrhage. Head injury may also disturb the regulation of cerebral and scalp vessels in a way that is still not fully understood.

There are many aspects of head injury which do not relate to our problem of headache. We are concerned with the patient who has experienced a head injury which may or may not have knocked him or her unconscious, who then recovers completely without any obvious damage to the nervous system, and yet who complains of frequent headaches which he or she attributes to the injury. What part is played by a change in sensitivity of nerves and vessels from damage at the time of the accident? What part is due to the state of anxiety and depression which often follows an accident, particularly one involving the head? Finally, what part can be blamed on the protracted litigation, which so often follows an accident, in attempting to assess whether the symptoms are the result of the accident and whether an insurance company or someone else has a financial liability?

THE SIZE OF THE PROBLEM

The incidence of post-traumatic headaches varies from 33 to 80 percent in various samplings. Doctor C. Brenner and his colleagues in Boston found that a headache lasting more than two months was uncommon in those patients who were only dazed but were not disoriented after the injury and in those who had little or no loss of memory for the period immediately following the injury (post-traumatic amnesia). The incidence of headache was higher in those patients whose scalp was lacerated. It was also higher in those who had a basically nervous disposition, those with symptoms of anxiety after the accident, and those with occupational difficulties or with pending litigation. Neither the time the patient was unconscious nor the existence of a skull fracture seemed to have any correlation with headache.

CONCUSSION

An individual who loses consciousness for a minute or two after a blow on the head and then recovers is said to have been concussed. The mechanism is still not completely understood, but it is clearly related to the movement of the brain within the skull. If the skull is crushed by some action without movement of the head —for example a car sliding off a hydraulic jack, so that part of it rests on the head of the mechanic—the skull may be fractured while the patient remains conscious. A small missile may penetrate the skull without consciousness being impaired. On the other hand, if a person is moving at 30 miles an hour or more and his skull hits a telephone pole, the skull decelerates instantaneously to zero. The brain continues to move in relation to the skull until it, too, decelerates to zero. Apart from causing direct damage to the surface of the brain, the sliding movement of the brain exerts a twisting action on the brain-stem which is relatively fixed in position. The center for maintaining the brain in a state of awareness is situated in the upper part of the brain-stem, in the line of maximum stress. The strain of the impact thus gives a "knock-out" blow to this vital center so that consciousness is lost.

Some minutes after regaining consciousness it is quite common for the individual to complain of a throbbing headache, which is worse on jarring or moving the head. The majority of people admitted to a hospital with concussion do not complain of headache in the immediate period after injury. Doctors O. N. Tubbs and J. M. Potter of The Radcliffe Infirmary, Oxford, England, found that some 60 percent did not experience headache at all while in the hospital, and only 11 percent complained spontaneously of headache or required analgesics for it. How and why then do headaches arise some days or weeks after the injury?

The early treatment of concussion may be important in reducing the disability which so often follows. A group of neurosurgeons from Helsinki contrasted the results of an active treatment program with the routine treatment of comparable patients in the same hospital. The active treatment group were visited daily, and the nature of the injury was explained to them. They were encouraged to get up out of bed and start physiotherapy. When they attended the follow-up clinic, they were seen by the same doctor who had looked after them in the hospital. The active treatment group returned to work in an average of eighteen days compared with thirty-two for the others. It is common experience that recovery from a football or other sporting injury is much more rapid and complete than after a traffic accident or an injury at work. The desire for monetary compensation is not the only factor involved in this. The force involved in the latter forms of head injury is usually much greater than blows acquired on the sporting field.

PROGRESSIVE HEADACHE AFTER INJURY

Every now and again one reads a small paragraph in a newspaper describing a schoolboy who was knocked unconscious for a few minutes while playing football, then sent to bed at home or boarding school apparently recovered, and found dead in bed the next morning. The reason for such tragedies is that the meningeal arteries which lie in the skull may bleed if a fracture line runs across them. Even without a fracture, veins which bridge the gap between the surface of the brain and the inner wall of the skull may be torn and bleed while the subject is completely unaware of it. The onset of headache within minutes or hours of a head injury must cause concern if it becomes progressively worse or if the patient also becomes drowsy. A hemorrhage of this kind may develop between the skull bone and the dura which lines it (extradural hematoma) or under the dural membrane (subdural hematoma). In either event it expands, compressing the brain, displacing vessels, and causing headache. The condition requires immediate neurosurgical attention so the clot can be removed and the pressure relieved.

A slow-motion subdural hemorrhage may cause trouble weeks or months after a head blow, which may have been so mild as to be forgotten by the time the headache starts. The headache progressively becomes worse and may be associated with drowsiness in a manner similar to that described for cerebral tumor. The important thing is to be aware of the possibility. Surgical treatment is easy once the diagnosis is made.

VASCULAR HEADACHES

Once we have excluded cerebral compression from an expanding clot, we are left with a variety of headaches. These are often grouped together with giddiness and anxiety symptoms in the postconcussional or posttraumatic syndrome. Doctor Harold G. Wolff considered that there were three main causes of headache in this syndrome. The first was a form of chronic muscle contraction or tension headache, the second was a local ache caused by scar tissue at the site of injury, and the third was a vascular headache resembling migraine. The latter was often one-sided and associated with nausea, vomiting, and distension of the scalp arteries in the manner of migraine. It is probable that any blow to or laceration of the scalp arteries renders them more liable to the painful dilatation that gives rise to posttraumatic migraine. The area of pain may be limited to a particular vessel in the forehead, temple, or back of the head in the part which was struck at the time of the injury. Sometimes a scar may be seen to traverse one of the major scalp arteries. Jabbing pains may also be felt at the site of a scar where nerves have been involved in the scar tissue. An operation to tie off and cut the affected artery (and nerve as well if it is involved too) often gives relief. Otherwise the treatment is the same as for migraine. Jabbing nerve pains usually respond well to medication with carbamazepine.

In addition to the migrainous pattern of headache, there is another form of vascular headache that may be caused by dilatation of the intracranial vessels and made worse by vasodilator agents such as histamine. It is frequently found in conjunction with muscle contraction headaches after head injury and is made worse by exertion.

WHIPLASH INJURY

The dramatic term "whiplash injury" conjures up a vision of the patient's neck being cracked like a whip —imagery more vivid than is usually warranted by the circumstances. The very use of the term may be enough to make the patient retract his neck like a tortoise, causing the neck muscles to contract continuously, a potent cause of headache in its own right. In any accident where the body is stabilized and the head is free to move, some degree of whiplash must take place. The classical example is the driver in a stationary car which is hit in the rear by another vehicle. The front car is pushed forward, the driver's back is pressed against the seat, and his head is forced backward. The reverse situation may occur when the driver of the moving car is wearing a seat belt which restrains his body at the moment when his car collides with another, so that his head flexes violently forward on the neck.

Immediately after such a collision the neck may feel stiff and sore and pain may occur in the back of the head. Mercifully, these symptoms usually disappear after a few days of discomfort and all is well again. When pain persists, it is often difficult to assess objectively, as X rays of the neck usually show no recent abnormality, and judgment must be made entirely on clinical grounds. Pain may radiate down to shoulders and arms or up to the back of the head and even to the forehead. There may be local tenderness in the neck or back of the skull. The pain can be derived from a displacement of part of the substance of a disk which lies between two vertebral bodies as a shock absorber (Figures 1,2). Pain can also arise from the interpedicular joints of the vertebrae, from the ligaments and soft tissues of the neck, or from stretching of nerve roots.

The condition may be treated by the injection of local anesthetic agents and hydrocortisone or long-acting steroids into the tender areas. It may also require immobilization of the neck by a plastic collar. The application of local heat and traction to the neck by a physiotherapist is often helpful. There are those who advocate manipulation of the neck, but this should be done only by those experienced in its use because there is potential danger that disk substance may be forced onto the spinal cord. This can cause complete paralysis of the legs, severe weakness of the arms, and loss of bladder and bowel function.

Doctor James Cyriax of St. Thomas' Hospital, London, who has long practiced manipulation of the neck, stresses that it should be done without any anesthesia, with the patient lying on his back with his head over the end of a bed, so that traction can be exerted on the neck in the extended position while the manipulation is in progress. With these precautions, he has never seen any untoward effect and has achieved some remarkably beneficial results.

The factor of compensation neurosis or even frankly hysterical behavior can add to the problem in some cases. I recall one patient who walked perfectly normally while wearing a surgical collar. On every occa-

sion when the collar was removed he underwent weird
gyrations, flailing his arms and legs. Eventually he fell
to the floor. A collar may be good treatment for a while,
but it is not essential to maintain the upright posture
and should not be allowed to take the place of the neck
muscles permanently.

MUSCULAR CONTRACTION

Doctor Harold Wolff examined a group of sixty-three
patients with chronic post-traumatic headache and recorded the electrical activity in the muscles of the scalp
and neck. He found that the muscles were continuously
active in three-quarters of the patients for the duration
of their headache. In twenty-eight of the thirty-seven
examined during a headache the muscle activity was
greatest at the site of the headache. This does not mean
that excessive muscle contraction is necessarily the sole
cause of the headache, but it must be an important
factor, since mental and physical relaxation may reduce
or eliminate the headache. This process is discussed in
greater detail in the next chapter.

The quality of muscle contraction headache is usually
a dull pressure sensation or tightness in the head. The
pressure is fairly continuous but fluctuates in intensity,
occasionally flaring up to a more painful throbbing
when vascular dilatation is superimposed. The sufferers
are usually tense, anxious, fretful, and often depressed.
They may also be resentful about the accident, about
the legal implications, and possibly also about the treatment they have or have not received from their doctors. All of this may be reinforced if they are referred
from doctor to doctor for opinions. The patient may
end up as a nobody's baby. The treatment is similar to
that for tension headache (described in the next chap-

ter), but it depends for its success on some doctor taking a personal and enduring interest in the patient's welfare.

TUMOR AND TRAUMA

Head injuries are very common, and brain tumors are rare. Nevertheless, an association has been claimed between head injury and the later development, up to thirty years afterward, of a meningioma, a benign tumor growing from the membranes of the skull. The association was first noted by the famous neurosurgeon, Dr. Harvey Cushing of Johns Hopkins Hospital, Baltimore; in 30 percent of his three hundred patients with meningioma, the tumor developed at the site of previous damage to the skull. This contention is hard to prove statistically, but it has been supported by the experience of many authors, including Sir Francis Walshe, who concluded "the perpetually open mind is not an effective instrument of thought, and may too easily become a euphemism for the mind closed to the lessons of experience."

COMPENSATION AND LITIGATION

If the persistence of symptoms after head injury were due to a conscious or subconscious desire for financial gain, it might be assumed that they would be present less often in those whose injury was not compensable and would disappear once the case was settled in the patient's favor. Neither of these suppositions is invariably correct. It used to be said by cynics that the cure for the post-traumatic syndrome is the insertion of gold into the palm of the hand. But is this the cure? Doctors John Balla and S. Moraitis from Melbourne followed up eighty-two patients of Greek extraction after they had been in industrial or traffic accidents which caused injuries to their necks and backs. Forty-one of them complained of bilateral headaches radiating up from the neck like a pressure sensation. Although original injuries were mild and many of the patients' symptoms were considered to have a psychological basis, the correlation between early settlement of the legal case and return to work was not high. At the time of settlement, forty had already gone back to work and eleven did so shortly afterward. But thirty-one patients continued to have symptoms which prevented them from working, even after the case had been decided and financial compensation awarded.

The facts that symptoms disappear in some patients who return to work before settlement of claims and persist in others after compensation has been agreed upon should not be allowed to disguise the fact that some patients do lack any motivation to return to work and that others have quite bizarre psychological reactions toward their injury and its legal aspects.

NEUROTIC OR ORGANIC?

Controversy still rages over the degree to which symptoms which follow head injury are determined by the medico-legal aspects, by a psychological reaction to injury, or by some subtle organic change. Some of the symptoms of anxiety and depression following head injury have already been mentioned. Doctor John Ellard of Sydney describes other patients in whom schizophrenia with paranoid ideas, hysterical conversion reactions, and hypochondriasis have been precipitated by head injury.

One of my own patients underwent a complete personality change after being knocked unconscious while working in a mine. His workmates mistakenly elected to drive him to the nearest hospital by car although he was still unconscious. He was supported in the sitting position, which reduced the blood supply to his concussed brain. After apparent physical recovery from his injury, he had changed from being a reliable, steady worker to a shiftless, evasive character with grossly hysterical behavior. He stated that he was unable to feel pain and demonstrated this by stubbing cigarette butts out on his arm or leg. Pathological changes have been observed in nerve cells as a result of brain concussion, and it seems reasonable to assume that in some patients these could account for an alteration in personality. Certainly some patients can never perform again at their previous level.

Whether or not minute changes in the structure of brain cells also play a part in the symptoms of anxiety and depression which are so frequent after head injury remains open to question. The self-employed return to work earlier on the average than those who are employed by others. This may be a question of motivation, but could also be related to the greater physical exertion required of employees in many industries, especially semiskilled workers and laborers—exertion which might make certain persistent symptoms intolerable.

There is good evidence that the giddiness which commonly follows head injury is caused by damage to that part of the inner ear concerned with the sense of balance. It may well be that many of the other symptoms have their basis in some form of damage which we are unable to detect by present methods. This is the view put forward by Dr. Alex R. Taylor, a neurosurgeon from Belfast in Northern Ireland. He says "Prima facie, it seems strange that 66 percent of the head-injured, necessarily a random sample of the population, should be afflicted with neuroticism or excessive cupidity while most of the victims of limb, abdominal, or thoracic injury escape these stigmata. The evidence for neuroticism should be carefully examined."

On the other side of the ledger, writers such as Professor Henry Miller of Newcastle-upon-Tyne have presented a case for the multitude of symptoms being a purely psychological reaction to the accident. He found that the majority of his patients did lose their symptoms after legal settlement. Only two out of fifty unselected patients were still disabled two years after settlement. The most that other patients could muster were a few trivial residual symptoms, such as "a queer feeling as I turn on the vacuum cleaner" and "some nervousness on overtaking in traffic." Miller concludes: "It seems clear that accident neurosis is not a function of the accident itself, but of the setting in which this occurred. In my opinion it is not a result of the accident but a concomitant of the compensation situation and a manifestation of the hope of financial gain." He makes a point which emphasizes the paradox in the treatment of this problem. "Doctor and lawyer are sometimes at cross-purposes over the question of settlement, the lawyer insisting that there should be no settlement without clinical finality, the doctor that there can be no clinical finality without settlement."

A BALANCED VIEW

Arguments have been presented for both sides of the case—are the symptoms psychological or organic? Considering that the mind is the product of the brain, the gap between these arguments may be narrowed.

We recognize extracranial vascular headaches similar to migraine resulting from damage to scalp vessels, and a less clearly defined intracranial vascular headache which may be made worse by exertion. This suggests that the very fact of a sudden acceleration or deceleration of the head may be sufficient to render cranial blood vessels more susceptible to painful dilatation. We recognize aching in the back of the head as related to disturbance of the upper neck. Above all, we concede the importance of excessive muscle contraction, alone or in combination with the other causes in maintaining the headache pattern, often after the initial structural damage has subsided.

The anxiety and depression which accompany muscle contraction seem to be related to the accident initially, although litigation worries may later aggravate the situation. The patient is naturally fearful that he will never be quite the same as before and that his capacity for work may be impaired. There is also a dread of another accident. I was once the victim of an explosion which caused extensive burns to my face and arm, and I well recall that my startle responses to any sudden sound were exaggerated for some weeks or months afterward. An extreme example of this fear was described by Ellard. A woman who had been involved in an automobile accident could only tolerate being driven by her husband if she could huddle under a rug on the floor in the back of the car drinking brandy. Problems like this require sympathetic understanding and psychotherapy.

Finally, there are always those who regard an accident as being a gift from the gods, a ticket in a lottery which may win them a substantial prize if they can hang on to the ticket long enough.

It requires an unbiased approach on the part of the

doctor, a careful assessment of each patient's personality and headache pattern, and a considerable degree of skill to ensure that justice is done to the patient's legal claim and that treatment is appropriate to the variety of headache.

7

Is Tension Headache All in the Mind?

The advertising world does not hesitate to suggest possible reasons and remedies for tension headaches. We usually are shown a stress situation such as a driver trapped in a traffic jam. The message is spelled out clearly: "Don't share your day with a headache." The remedy appears to be simple: "Take several pills of 'Brand X' and your headache will disappear." In fact, this often does prove to be the case. Most of us are subject to headaches on the odd occasion when there is unusual pressure at home or work, or we are enduring a period of frustration, or suffering from glare combined with heat. No one could object to the taking of analgesic tablets to get rid of these particular types of headache. If the headaches recur frequently, even daily, and the consumption of analgesics creeps up steadily, the problem becomes more serious and requires medical attention. The continued daily use of analgesic tablets is a common cause of serious kidney disease in later life.

TENSION, ANYONE?

Confusion exists about the meaning of the word tension in the context of tension headache. Does it mean that the patient is aware of inner tensions of emotional or mental origin, of some conflict between pleasure and duty, or some situation in his or her personal life that has no possible solution? Or does it mean a state of physical tension which prevents the body from relaxing in the absence of perceptible emotional problems? We might reasonably expect the two to go together, and yet curiously enough we frequently encounter one without the other.

Some people may survive the most incredible succession of irritations, frustrations, or personal tragedies without their mental state being reflected in bodily symptoms, possibly because they surrender themselves to the situation, accept their inability to alter it, and swim with the current. Others faced with the same type of situation suppress their emotional reactions, keep their sadness, resentment, or aggression to themselves, and attempt to battle the current. The burdens of life lie unevenly on people's shoulders, not only those burdens which may eventually be remedied by economic, social, or humanitarian measures, but also those imposed by blind fate. Individuals vary greatly in their ability to bear their burden, light or heavy. There must be few of us, indeed, who are not subject to stress at

The Wizard of Id

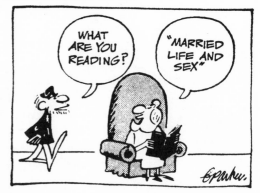

some time or other. Some who have no burden to carry often seek one, real or imagined. Mental stress leads to physical stress. The combination is known as nervous tension, one symptom of which is tension headache.

A word about the meaning of hypertension. Some patients are under the impression that hypertension is a sort of superstress. "I am not only in a state of tension, I have hypertension." The medical meaning of hypertension is more prosaic, simply meaning a blood pressure which is higher than the normal range. Blood pressure does increase in situations of nervous tension, but the terms "tension" and "hypertension" are used to denote entirely different sorts of pressures.

CHARACTERISTICS OF TENSION HEADACHE

We are not concerned here with the occasional headache but with headaches which recur several times each month, several times each week, or every day.

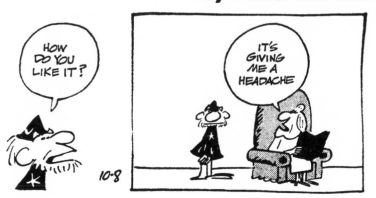

This is called chronic tension headache. In our experience of patients attending a headache clinic, the condition is almost as common as migraine.

Of 1,152 patients seen in our clinic over a period of two and one-half years with the complaint of chronic headache, 612 suffered from migraine and 466 from tension headache. Some 15 percent of the patients with tension headache remember their symptoms starting before the age of ten, so this can be quite a problem in children as well as in adults. As is the case with migraine, 75 percent of patients with tension headache are women. The condition may persist throughout life, and we have seen elderly patients who have experienced headache almost daily for fifty or sixty years. Why women should be more susceptible to tension headache than men remains a mystery. Women traditionally have shown their feelings more than men, but their emotional tone fluctuates more widely and they are generally more sensitive to minor frustrations or disappointments. This may be explicable by hormonal changes. Premenstrual tension symptoms are very common with irritability and depression accompanying the fall in hormonal levels at the end of the menstrual cycle. Estimations of hormones in the blood show a considerable variation from day to day and even at different times of the same day. It would not be surprising if emotional reactions altered in parallel with the swings in hormone levels. Hormones certainly influence regulation of blood vessels and are responsible for the higher incidence of migraine in women, but whether vascular reactivity is a factor in tension headache is uncertain.

Tension headache affects both sides of the head symmetrically in 90 percent of patients, unlike migraine which is usually felt mainly on one side of the head. The quality of the headache is remarkably consistent and characteristic. It is more of a tightness, a constant feeling of pressure than a pain. It is described as a dull ache in the forehead, the temples, the back of the head, or "all over the head." It feels like a weight on the head, a constant heaviness, or a tight band around the head. Some patients also notice sudden jabs of pain on one side of the head, on the top of the head, or in the back of the head and neck, which are superimposed on a background of general discomfort. For approximately one-fourth of all patients, there are periods when the headache becomes more severe or throbbing in quality and the patient may feel nauseated. This change indicates that dilatation of blood vessels has become a factor in the production of pain. These "tension-vascular" headaches form a link with episodic headaches more typical of migraine. Some 10 percent of patients with tension headache are also subject to migraine. However, we cannot regard tension headache as a form of migraine. The number of close relatives who suffer from migraine is 45 percent in the case of migrainous patients, but only 18 percent for tension headache patients (no greater than the general population).

The patient subject to chronic tension headache experiences symptoms not only during a distasteful situation but may develop a headache in anticipation of any unpleasantness. Just before the battle with Tweedledee, Tweedledum remarked "I'm very brave generally, only today I happen to have a headache." The symptoms may later start to appear in advance of a normal day's work, a routine shopping expedition, a trip into town, a visit to friends, or any of the other trivial rituals of daily life. Then the headache may start to waken the patient from sleep, although it more often appears as he or she gets up and about, greeting each new day with a less than optimistic eye. It may be associated with other symptoms of nervous tension—a pain under the left breast, for example, or a sensation of tightness in the chest. The patient takes deep sighing breaths in an attempt to ease this feeling of tightness. A feeling of light-headedness, which is caused by washing carbon dioxide out of the lungs, often results. Underlying all the symptoms there is usually an inability to relax, a feeling of physical tension, and often a mild fluctuating depression. The patients rarely feel elated or exuberant and are usually content to suffer quietly, like the lugubrious character in an old radio comedy who kept repeating in sepulchral tones, "It's being so cheerful what keeps me going." In contrast to most other kinds of headache, tension headache is usually relieved by taking alcohol, a useful point in diagnosis. It is as though some people were "born two drinks down on life" and require that little bit of extra support from other sources to lift their emotional tone up to a normal level.

The outward appearance of a patient with tension headache may be bland, set, and expressionless, like a mask of forebearance. Or it may clearly show the lifetime habit of muscle contraction in a furrowed brow and deep-set facial lines. He or she may continually clutch a handkerchief to disguise his or her sweating palms and may wear dark glasses, however gloomy the day outside. This seems a caricature, but there is considerable truth in it. Exceptional patients may smile gaily while describing the constant aching that makes life intolerable for them.

MUSCLE CONTRACTION AS THE MECHANISM OF TENSION HEADACHE

Tension headache is *not* all in the mind. There is no question of it being imaginary. There *is* a tightness and aching in the forehead, the temples, or the back of the head. There may also be a sensation of a constant pressure in the neck and jaws. The feeling of pressure on the top of the head can come from a sheet of fibrous tissue which stretches over the top of the skull, to which are attached the scalp muscles. If the scalp muscles constantly contract, they pull on this fibrous sheet and maintain tension on it. Pressure sensations or aching is associated with constant overcontraction of the muscles of the jaws, face, and neck. Doctor Harold G. Wolff and his colleagues recorded the electrical activity of these muscles and were able to correlate the pain sensation with the degree of muscle contraction. They found that the major scalp arteries tended to constrict at the time of tension headache, whereas they dilate in migraine and other vascular headaches. They put forward the hypothesis that the scalp and adjacent muscles were working overtime with less than the normal blood supply to sustain them. This would explain the known action of warmth, massage, and vasodilator agents, including alcohol, in relieving tension headache, since all of these improve the blood supply to the scalp. They also found that the pain subsided when the muscles were infiltrated with a local anesthetic, indicating that the pain originated from the muscles. Some patients whose vessels are constricted all day may undergo a rebound dilatation at night and thus awaken in the early hours of the morning with a tension-vascular headache.

It is a common observation that chronic frowners

tend to have their headache in the forehead, that the jaw-clenchers complain of headache in the temples where the jaw-closing muscles are attached to the bone, and that the "stiff-necks" who walk around with their head held rigidly notice pain in the back of the head and in the neck. Why doesn't everyone who frowns get tension headache? Perhaps the answer lies in the vascular changes that Wolff observed, by the accumulation of pain-producing substances in areas where the blood is inadequate to supply the contracting muscles. Tension headache tends to run in families since some 40 percent of close relatives complain of similar symptoms. The distribution of muscular activity can often be seen particularly well in an electroencephalogram and may help to confirm the diagnosis. The electrical activity of muscle contraction is quite different from that of the brain and may be detected in the recording, usually overlying the site where the patient complains of pain. There are some other physical factors which may aggravate the tendency to muscle contraction and which must be considered in the treatment process.

AGGRAVATING FACTORS

Eyestrain.   A tension headache may be set up by the effort required to overcome imbalance of the eye muscles or other forms of defective vision. These aspects should be checked by an ophthalmologist if the headache consistently follows prolonged reading.

Neck posture.   If a child is required to sit at a desk in a chair which is too low or too high, he must crane his neck muscles constantly to see books clearly, to write, or to view the chalkboard. Childrens' furniture has to be adjusted from time to time as they grow. The penalty for failing to do so is pain in the head and neck. The same sort of situation applies to the drivers of cars who accommodate their posture to the car instead of finding a car which has seats suitable for them.

If there is a disturbance of the bones, disks, ligaments, or muscles of the neck which becomes painful or which makes an occasional crunching noise (more alarming than harmful), a secondary muscle contraction headache is almost inevitable. Treatment must be directed at the primary cause in the neck.

Jaw-clenching and fang-sharpening. Imbalance of the bite caused by loss of back teeth on one side or the other or by ill-fitting dentures can set up a faulty habit of jaw-clenching and tooth-grinding. Dental attention is obviously a prerequisite for successful treatment. I have known patients to fracture one set of dentures after another because of their persistent habit of jaw-clenching and others who have had to have most of their teeth recapped because their continual tooth-grinding had worn the enamel away.

Doctor R. G. Every, a dental surgeon from New Zealand, considers gnashing the teeth to be a signal of aggressive behavior, grinding the teeth as symbolic of sharpening weapons of aggression, and clenching the jaws as a means of protecting these weapons. His thesis maintains that when man is under stress, he will sharpen his teeth: "To prepare for an emergency he grinds his teeth together—innately and unconsciously." Doctor Every drew attention to lateral movements of the jaw which can take place during the "fang-sharpening" process in sleep. He has pointed out that some people may awaken with a bruised area inside the mouth as a result of these nocturnal movements. I have certainly had complaints from a patient's wife or husband that their spouse keeps them awake by the clashing of tooth on tooth in the night. I have also seen

patients with the sore areas in the mouth described
by Every. Whether the evolutionary explanation is correct or not, the possibility of repressed aggression
must be considered, and underlying anxiety must be
treated.

The mental background. While the physical cause
of tension headache, or muscle contraction headache,
as it is often called, is fairly well established, the underlying mental or emotional conflict remains unresolved
in the majority of patients. Doctor Arnold P. Friedman
of New York and his associates considered that the most
common factors were a repressed hostility toward the
family, resentment of authority, the need to inhibit sexual temptation, and the unconscious wish to remain in
a position of dependence in order to obtain attention,
affection, and love. Doctors Martin, Rome, and Swenson of the Mayo Clinic found that the conflicts described by patients were associated with anxiety, anger,
or frustration. Specific problems were difficulty in leaving home, passive submission to a domineering spouse,
broken marriages, sexual problems (such as impotence,
premature ejaculation, or frigidity), a poor work record,
and emotional disturbances, particularly depression.
Some patients literally described members of the
family as "a pain in the neck." No special "headache
personality" was found. It appears that muscle contraction headache represents a psychophysiological expression of anxiety whatever the cause.

It is incorrect to think of patients with chronic tension headache as necessarily having an inadequate personality. It may well be that a well-motivated person's
relentless drive that has made him a success in his
chosen field has also made him prey to the equally
relentless overactivity of his own musculature. Finally,
I must say that many of my patients do not appear to

have any present problem which can be defined as unresolved conflict. They simply have a habit of muscular contraction which has been with them through an otherwise untroubled life.

PSYCHOLOGICAL TREATMENT

The treatment of tension headache requires a holistic approach to the patient and his or her problems when these can be identified. It is first necessary to explain the mechanism of tension headache and the important part played by muscle contraction. The patient must feel completely reassured about the absence of cerebral tumor or other organic disturbance. Otherwise he or she will move from doctor to doctor, from doctor to chiropractor, from chiropractor to acupuncturist, and somewhere along the line the patient may receive part of the answer, part of the support and reassurance he or she is seeking.

Some patients benefit from a discussion with their doctor of immediate or long-standing problems, without the need for formal psychotherapy. It is remarkable what profound feelings may have been repressed for so long, simply for want of some understanding yet authoritative figure to whom patients can unburden themselves. Many such anxieties are of sexual origin— long repressed fears about masturbation, guilt about premarital intercourse or later infidelity, anxiety about the possibility of venereal disease being acquired in the past (almost invariably groundless), or unvoiced feelings of homosexuality. It took a number of interviews before a middle-aged man confessed that his life had been tarnished by a long-standing belief that masturbation in adolescence had been responsible for his penis remaining undersized. He had always avoided sporting activities and changing rooms because of the fear that other men would notice the size of his penis and associate it with his clandestine masturbation. He was not helped by the one person in whom he had confided in all these years who said, "Well, perhaps that *is* the reason." When reassured that masturbation was almost universal among adolescent boys, and that the size of his penis was well within the normal range, and that there was no possible connection between the two, his whole attitude changed. His headache disappeared as though a cloud had been lifted and he said, "Why couldn't I have been told this thirty years ago?" The reassurance that many experiences are quite normal can give great relief to someone who has always regarded his or her particular problem as unique. Sexual counseling by a physician or psychiatrist skilled in this field can be of enormous assistance, particularly for specific problems such as impotence and premature ejaculation in men and frigidity in women.

Advice may also be required about the handling of everyday life situations. The following simple rules are taken from *Psychosomatic Medicine* by Edward Weiss and O. Spurgeon English of Philadelphia:

1. This is not a perfect world. Families and friends, too, have their failings. Perfection is rarely attained, so be satisfied with less.
2. Tolerance makes understanding the other fellow easier. It sets an attainable standard.
3. Do not be a slave to the clock. Work at your own pace. Do as much as you can. Trying to meet too many deadlines only creates tension.
4. You cannot please everybody, so stop trying. Popularity comes by giving your friends and family a chance to love you for yourself, not for your best performance.

5. Be efficient, yes, but not to the extent that perfection becomes a burden.
6. Speak up if you want to. You cannot please everybody, and honesty and directness break down barriers and makes friendships easier.
7. Approve of yourself. You are as good as the next fellow.
8. Stop being so critical of your negative feelings. Everyone is ambivalent at times, so do not worry so much about loving and hating.
9. Stop feeling so guilty. We are all human beings, and we all make errors. Give a little and you will get a lot—maybe even a reduction of the pain in your head.

Explanation and advice about the style of life and its associated problems may be all that is required. However, some patients may benefit from formal psychotherapy, and some patients with severe depression or thought disorders are best referred to a psychiatrist as soon as this is recognized.

PHYSICAL AND PHARMACOLOGICAL TREATMENT

There are many patients whose problems are either inapparent or insoluble. Some of them say that they have not a care in the world apart from their headache, while others admit to persisting symptoms of anxiety and depression. The first step is for the patient to realize that the muscles of the face, scalp, and neck are contracting unnecessarily, the second for the patient to practice relaxation of one muscle group after the other. This concept is not new, but has never been employed on a large scale. Doctor Edmund Jacobsen of Chicago made notable early contributions to the subject, and there have since been other books which are also useful reading for anyone subject to tension headache. Based on the principles of these authors, a simple series of relaxation exercises for patients is suggested. The only basic difference between my recommendations and those of others is my emphasis on a positive attempt to relax, to "switch off" the muscle mechanisms. Ideally, the initial sessions should take place in the presence of an instructor who can ensure that the correct sequence is being carried out and that the subject is indeed relaxing correctly. More formal training in relaxation has been introduced in which electrodes are attached to skin over muscles to record the electrical activity set up by muscular contraction. This is amplified and played back through a loudspeaker so that the patient can hear a sound which varies in intensity with the degree of muscle contraction. He can then practice relaxation until the sound disappears. This is known as a "feedback technique," because information is fed back to the participant.

There are some patients who may lose their headaches as the result of relaxation exercises alone, just as there are some who may respond to psychotherapy alone. I personally find it helpful to prescribe a relaxant pill such as diazepam in the initial stages or to use an antidepressant such as amitriptyline if the patient has an underlying depression. The object of pharmacotherapy is to free the patient of headache as soon as possible and then to take him or her off the medication slowly, as soon as the relaxation process is well established. I find this a useful way of breaking the vicious circle of analgesic intake, which leads to rebound headaches in the short term and to serious kidney damage if continued long term. This is a matter that each patient must discuss with his or her doctor because each doctor will have his or her own view about the desirability of medication, the type of medication, and the length of time it should be continued. The response in some patients placed on relaxant or antidepressant therapy can be quite dramatic. Some patients find that their heads feel clear for the first time in ten, twenty, or thirty years. It therefore has an important place but is no substitute for correction of the underlying mental and physical causes.

ARE YOU ABLE TO RELAX?

The blood vessels and nerve fibers of the scalp lie in muscle. Place your fingers on each temple and clench your jaw. You will feel the temporal muscle swell as it contracts. Let the jaw go loose and the muscle becomes flat again. Many people contract these muscles all day without realizing it, so they are working continuously. This sets up a constant dull ache in the temples. Do you feel the jaw muscles aching at the end of the day, or after an unpleasant or difficult conversation, or after an argument? Do you feel an ache in one or both temples at these times, or do you wake up with a headache in this area?

Just as chronic jaw-clenching is a common cause of aching in the temples, chronic frowning is a common cause of pain in the forehead. Do others say to you that you frown a lot or look worried most of the time? This can be an indication that you are using your scalp muscles without being aware of it. Pain in the neck can also result from muscle contraction. Some people walk about holding their necks stiffly as though they were solid blocks of wood. Overcontraction of muscle is a faulty habit which develops over the years and often starts in childhood. It may be associated with mental tension and anxiety but may also have become an automatic reaction that continues even when there are no problems.

The most natural form of treatment is training the muscles of the body to relax. The first step is to realize that you are not as relaxed as you think you are.

Try these simple tests:

1. Sit in a chair and lean back. Ask someone to lift your arm in the air into a comfortable position as though it were resting on the side of an arm chair. Take your time and relax completely. Then ask your friend to take away his or her hands which have been supporting your arm. When the supporting hands are taken away, what does your arm do?

   If it flops lifelessly downward, you are indeed relaxed. If it stays in the air, or you move it slowly downward, you are not relaxed. Your muscles are contracting continuously *without your realizing it.*

2. Lie on a bed or couch with your head on a pillow and try to relax completely. When you consider that you have achieved this, ask your associate to pull the pillow away from under your head.

   Does your head drop limply onto the bed? Or does it stay poised in midair as though the pillow were still there?

   If you are still holding your head in the air above an invisible pillow, your muscles must be contracting *without your realizing it.*

Once you have acknowledged that excessive muscle contraction is playing a part in the aching of your head or neck and that you do not really know whether the muscles are contracting or not, you are ready to start relaxation exercises.

Paradoxically, you cannot relax about relaxing. It is not a passive process. It is no use saying to someone,

"Relax," and imagine that they can do it without further thought. You cannot say to yourself, "Relax," and then do it unless you have carefully practiced the art of "switching off" the nerve supply to the muscles. This is a voluntary action as deliberate as turning off a light switch and must be practiced until it can be done at will and done quickly.

At first it is necessary to set aside at least ten minutes night and morning for the exercises. It is a great help to have someone with you in the early stages to ensure that you are completely relaxed when you think you are. This person will be referred to below as the "assistant." It is obviously a great advantage if the assistant can be a trained physiotherapist or occupational therapist, but this is not always practicable, and a well-motivated companion can be of enormous value in ensuring that the exercises are performed conscientiously and that relaxation is practiced until it becomes complete.

THE SEQUENCE OF RELAXATION EXERCISES

Lie down on a firm surface such as a carpeted floor. A bed with an inner-spring mattress will do, but not one with a soft, sagging mattress. A pillow can be used to support the head at first but may be discarded later as relaxation becomes easier. For the first few sessions a short-sleeved shirt and shorts should be worn so that muscle contraction can be seen as well as felt. Lie on the back with the legs slightly separated and the arms comfortably flexed at the elbows so that the elbows are by the sides with the hands resting on the body. Various muscles will be contracted and relaxed in turn.

1. *Legs.* Contract the leg muscles so that the legs become rigid. The muscles will be seen to stand out as they contract. Concentrate on the sensation set up by the muscles contracting and the feeling of tension in them. Then, suddenly and deliberately, "switch off the power supply" so that the muscles become limp. Concentrate on whether any sensation is coming from the muscles now. Are they completely relaxed? At this point it is helpful for an assistant to put his or her hand behind the subject's knees and lift them up sharply to see if the leg is completely floppy and that the muscles do not contract again as soon as the limb is moved passively. If they are not completely relaxed or if they contract again when the limb is touched or moved, the sequence should be repeated. Many people only half-relax on the first few attempts. This can be detected by watching the muscles closely. After the first relaxation, the muscles are not as prominent as they were, but there may be some contraction remaining. Try again to "switch off," and this second attempt may be rewarded by seeing the muscle become completely flaccid. The legs may then be bent at the knee by the assistant, moved about, or rolled backward and forward with the feet flailing "like a rag doll." This sequence may be completed by lifting one leg, letting it drop downward like an inanimate object, then doing the same with the other.

2. *Arms.* Brace the arms so that the elbows are forced downward on the couch (or on the assistant's hand if he or she is checking the degree of relaxation). The arms are held rigidly, and the muscle contraction is suddenly stopped so that the arms become limp and lifeless. The assistant should then be able to bounce the elbow up and down without any resistance being offered. This sequence should

be repeated until the subject is aware of the sensation of muscle contraction and a contrast with the
feeling of relaxation and the assistant is satisfied
that the arm has become flaccid.

3. *Neck.* Lift the head from the pillow and then allow it to drop backward. The assistant may provide
resistance by pressing on the forehead until the
subject feels the contraction of the muscles in the
front of the neck. When the head is dropped backward, the assistant can rock it gently to and fro to
make certain that there is no residual activity in the
muscles. Now push the head backward into the pillow and register the sensation of contraction of the
muscles in the back of the neck. Stop the contraction suddenly so that the head may be rotated
freely on the neck by the assistant. Repeat this until
relaxation is satisfactory.

4. *Forehead.* Frown upward so that the brow is furrowed. If there is difficulty in doing this, look upward as far as the eyes will move until the forehead
becomes creased. Again, feel the sensation of tension in the muscles, then close the eyes and let the
forehead muscles relax. The assistant can detect the
presence or absence of contraction by seeing
whether the skin of the forehead moves freely with
his hand.

5. *Eyes.* Screw the eyes up tightly and become
aware of the sensation of tension, then relax the
muscles and lie with the eyes closed lightly. Make
sure that there is no trembling or flickering of the
closed eyelids and that the eye muscles feel entirely
relaxed.

6. *Jaw.* Clench the jaw firmly and concentrate on
feeling the sense of tightness in the temples as well
as in the jaw itself. Then switch off and let the jaw
loll open. Push the jaw open, perhaps against the
pressure of the assistant's hand, then relax com-

pletely. Move the jaw sideways to the right as far as
it will go and experience the sensation which this
gives to the jaw and temple before relaxing. Then
do the same to the left. Complete the sequence by
clenching the jaw firmly again, and let the jaw drop
open loosely. The assistant should then be able to
hold the tip of the jaw with his or her fingers and
waggle the jaw up and down rapidly without any
opposition from the jaw muscles.

This is the hardest of all relaxation procedures to
achieve and you must not be disappointed if you
are unsuccessful on the first occasion. It may require repeated practice to enable the jaw muscles
to cease all activity so that the jaw may be moved
easily by the assistant. It is most important that you
persevere until you accomplish this because overcontraction of jaw muscles is the most common factor in tension headache and the "switching-off"
process must be thoroughly learned.

7. *Whole body relaxation.* Once you are able to
relax the legs, arms, neck, forehead, eye, and jaw
muscles in that order, lie for five minutes with all
muscles relaxed. When you have achieved total
relaxation, the process becomes negative rather
than positive. In other words, you permit natural
relaxation to continue rather than willing yourself
to relax. At this stage, it is helpful to think of some
beautiful and tranquil scene, to imagine yourself
lying on a grassy bank on a warm summer's day
with the drowsy sounds of summer in the background. Everyone has some particular sound he or
she associates with peace and tranquillity. It may be
the rippling of a trout stream, the humming of bees,
the song of birds, the sighing of wind in the trees,
or distant music. Choose your own theme and your
own mental picture and live in that scene for a few
minutes. As you do so, feel the sensation of heavi-

ness creep over your legs, trunk, and arms, then move up to your neck and head, eyes, and face. This can become a permanent freedom if your muscles obey you at other times as well as they are doing at this moment.

After relaxation exercises are finished

The final and most important step is to carry the art of relaxation into your everyday life. Watch the way you stand, the way you sit, the way you speak on the telephone, talk to people, write, type, or perform any other activity on a typical day. Check that all the muscles which are not essential to the task of the moment are in a state of relaxation. You can handle any situation, irrespective of the degree of mental stress, without physical tension once you become accustomed to the idea. You actually perform more efficiently if you tackle any problem in an orderly fashion without excessive and useless muscle contraction. If you notice any warning sensations of tension in the scalp, jaw, or neck muscles, you must pause a moment to ensure that these muscles are "switched off" in the manner you have practiced. In this way you will finish the day feeling much fresher and have much less chance of having a headache make your day a misery.

Keep practicing

There is no point in performing the exercise routine religiously for a week and then forgetting the whole thing. If you do, the old habits of muscle contraction will assert themselves again. Keep practicing, stay relaxed, and free yourself from tension headache.

8

What Is Migraine?

The word *migraine* is French and derives from the Greek *hemicrania,* meaning that the pain involves half of the head at one time. This is not necessarily the case, however, since about one-third of headaches which have all the other characteristics of migraine involve both sides of the head. Indeed, careful observations have shown that blood flow alters on both sides of the head even though the pain may be felt mainly on only one side.

CLASSIC AND COMMON MIGRAINE

The important point in the diagnosis of migraine is that the headache is episodic, recurring at intervals peculiar to each individual, and is usually associated with nausea, blurring of vision, and sensitivity to light and sound. About one-third of all patients also experience odd disturbances of the nervous system such as the sensation of flashing lights in front of the eyes, pins and needles spreading around the mouth, numbness creeping up the arms and legs, slurring of speech, or difficulty in choosing the correct word. These symptoms are caused by blood being shunted away from the cerebral cortex which is near the surface of the brain and contains the nerve cells responsible for perception, thought, and speech. The unique feature of migraine is that large arteries and veins dilate while the network of smaller vessels, which normally carry the blood from the arteries to the veins, is shut off by constriction (so that blood bypasses areas of the cerebral cortex). The cells, deprived of their normal blood supply, first become excited so that the person sees stars, flashes, or zigzags of light, or feels other extraordinary sensations. Next, the nerve cells become silent and inactive so that the migraine sufferer is unable to see one-half of objects, or to feel one side of the body normally, or to speak correctly. The same process also affects the vessels outside the skull so that the large arteries of the scalp pulsate strongly and veins may be seen to stand out on the temple or forehead. In spite of this dilatation of large vessels, the skin becomes pale because blood is shunted away from the skin.

The association of visual or other symptoms with severe paroxysmal headache is known as "classic migraine." If the headache recurs periodically without these cerebral symptoms, it is called "nonclassic" or "common" migraine. The distinction between the two terms is probably artificial. Doctor Erik Skinhøj from Copenhagen has recently shown that the same sort of changes in blood flow take place in both common and classic migraine and that some parts of the brain have a diminished blood supply even in common migraine.

While descriptions of migraine may be found in antiquity, the first records of real clinical value were written in the late eighteenth and nineteenth centuries with the writings of Fothergill (1778), Tissot (1834), Labarraque (1837), Marshall Hall (1849), Du Bois Reymond (1860), Möllendorf (1867), and the classic treatise *On Megrim, Sick-headache and Some Allied Disorders* by Edward Liveing in 1873.

Du Bois Reymond wrote about his own attacks of common migraine:

Since about my twentieth year, although otherwise in good health, I have suffered from migraine. Every three or four weeks I am liable to an attack, coming on for the most part in consequence of some unhealthy influence, such as long fasting, a fatiguing evening, entertainment, and so forth. As a general rule some constipation precedes it. I thereupon awake the next morning with a general feeling of disorder, and a slight pain in the region of the right temple, which, without overstepping the middle line, gradually extends itself, reaching its greatest intensity at mid-day; towards evening it usually passes off. While at rest the pain is bearable, but it is increased by motion to a high degree of violence. It is aggravated by every circumstance which heightens the pressure of blood in the head, as stooping and coughing. It responds to each beat of the temporal artery. The latter feels, on the affected side, like a hard cord, whilst the left is in its normal condition. The countenance is pale and sunken, the right eye small and reddened. At the height of the attack, when it is a violent one, there is nausea, but as far as I remember, it has only once occasioned vomiting. As the attack approaches its termination the right ear reddens and feels a lively sense of warmth, which is also perceptible to the hand. Sleep often shortens the attack considerably, which leaves behind it a slight gastric disorder; frequently, also, the scalp remains tender at one spot the following morning. For a certain period after an attack I can expose myself with impunity to certain injurious influences which before would have infallibly induced an attack.

Fothergill described the visual disturbances of classic migraine and was the first to use the term *fortification* to describe their zigzag appearance. "After breakfast, if much toast and butter has been used, it begins with a singular kind of glimmering in the sight; objects swiftly changing their apparent position, surrounded with luminous angles like those of a fortification. Giddiness then comes on with headache and sickness." Liveing gives a more vivid description: "It commences with a slight dimness of sight; then the lower half, rather inclined to one side, of the field of view appears as if hidden by some white (luminous?) object held close to the eye. Gradually a half ring formed by serrated lines of prismatic colours appears in the place of the blank whiteness, the alternate points seeming to revolve in opposite directions. In about three quarters of an hour or an hour, this appearance ceases, and a violent headache succeeds." Another patient of Liveing's "became conscious of spectral objects like sparks or bright beads in incessant motion in the circumference of the field. The motion was very rapid and difficult to describe, but it always reminded me of the effect produced by the rapid gyrations of the lesser water beetles as I have seen them in patches on rivers and ponds in the bright sunshine."

The division of migraine into classic and nonclassic marks both ends of the spectrum, but there are some patients whose symptoms are difficult to classify into one group or the other because their only cerebral symptoms may be loss of concentration, mental confusion, giddiness, or emotional disturbances. These are almost certainly caused by the same process as the easily recognizable visual and sensory experiences. Other patients may have headaches which are accompanied by cerebral symptoms at some stage of their lives but not at other times. It is obvious that the basic recurring disturbance is the same throughout life but that its manifestations differ, depending on the degree to which the scalp vessels and the cerebral vessels are involved at any one time.

VARIATIONS ON THE THEME OF MIGRAINE

Migraine equivalents

In most patients the cerebral symptoms which have been described last for some ten to thirty minutes, after which the headache appears. In others they develop or continue while the headache is in progress. In a few they may occur on their own without any headache ensuing. This is called a "migraine equivalent." It is not uncommon for classic migraine to recur intermittently throughout life until middle age when the headache component progressively lessens, leaving the cerebral symptoms as the only manifestation, like Lewis Carroll's Cheshire Cat which "vanished quite slowly, beginning with the end of the tail, and ending with the grin, which remained some time after the rest of it had gone."

Double vision (ophthalmoplegic migraine)

Weakness of the eye muscles causing double vision is not uncommon in migraine, but it is unusual for this to be accompanied by an obvious squint. The pupils may become unequal in migraine, but if one pupil becomes greatly dilated and eye movements are impaired, the condition is called ophthalmoplegic migraine, the term meaning paralysis of the eye muscles. While this condition is well recognized, it is important to exclude causes other than migraine that can cause these symptoms by pressure on the nerves behind the eye.

One-sided weakness (hemiplegic migraine)

Hemiplegia means weakness of one-half of the body. Some patients experience weakness of one arm and leg before or during migraine headache, with or without a feeling of numbness or pins and needles. If the right arm and leg are affected in a right-handed person, the power of speech may also be impaired so that words are jumbled and the meaning lost. This condition is called hemiplegic migraine and tends to run in families, sometimes as a dominant characteristic. In other words, roughly half of all children of an affected parent will develop the condition. When it happens for the first time, the sufferer is understandably frightened, thinking that he or she is about to have a stroke. The symptoms are indeed similar. A stroke is caused by an obstruction of the blood flow in the arteries feeding the brain, which robs part of the brain of its blood supply. The symptoms in migraine are caused by a temporary diversion of blood from the same parts of the brain. The weakness usually clears up in an hour or so but may persist for some days. It is extremely rare for the weakness to become permanent, but it may in the case of women who are subject to this particular form of migraine and who are placed on contraceptive pills. This is the only type of migraine that causes a doctor to advise that oral contraceptives never be prescribed.

Loss of balance, giddiness, and fainting (basilar migraine)

If the blood supply to the hind-brain (the brain-stem and rear part of the cerebral cortex) is affected by the migrainous spasm of small vessels, the symptoms may then include a feeling of instability and loss of balance and coordination in addition to the visual symptoms. The patient may feel giddy, sway to and fro, bump into objects, and drop things. His or her speech may thicken and become slurred so that the whole appearance suggests that the patient could be drunk. If the spasm of vessels is severe enough, the patient may faint. This form of migraine is encountered mainly in girls and

young women, but some of the symptoms may occur at
any age. The blood supply of the hind-brain comes from
the vertebral arteries via the basilar artery (see Figures
2, 4). The condition was therefore designated "basilar
artery migraine" by Dr. E. R. Bickerstaff in 1961. Most
patients with migraine have some of these hind-brain
symptoms, and it is likely that the basilar artery circulation is temporarily impaired in all cases.

Blindness in one eye (retinal migraine)

If the small arteries supplying the retina at the back
of the eye are constricted during the migraine attack,
visual hallucinations may be limited to one eye instead
of one-half of the field seen with each eye as it is when
the brain vessels are affected. Vision in that eye may be
lost partly or completely for some minutes. As it recovers, a dull ache usually develops behind that eye and
may spread to the rest of the head.

Abdominal migraine

It is very common for children to have attacks of
vomiting whenever a party or other excitement is in
the offing. Some parents avoid telling their children of
any plans until the last moment because they know that
a "bilious attack" will surely develop. This condition is
recognized as a forerunner of migraine in later life.
Doctor Michael Anthony and I found that about a quar-
ter of our adult patients with migraine had been troubled with recurrent vomiting attacks in childhood.
Careful questioning of many of these children discloses
that they do have some sort of headache accompanying vomiting attacks. Some also have pain in the abdomen.

Whether recurring abdominal pain can be a form of
migraine, if there is no associated headache, nausea, or

vomiting, remains uncertain. There are a few documented cases where typical visual symptoms have been followed by abdominal pain and nausea without headache, which appear to be variations on the theme of migraine.

OTHER SYMPTOMS ASSOCIATED WITH MIGRAINE

A familiar story among migraine sufferers is that they can predict when an attack is coming. They feel a curious exhilaration the day before—they are "on top of the world." An unfortunate aftermath of the attack is that the patient may feel depressed, exhausted, and miserable for several days. In some patients, the sequence is reversed so that they feel irritable and depressed before the attack and in a particularly good mood when it ceases.

Many people have experienced distortions of vision or bodily sensations when dropping off to sleep or lying in bed only half-awake. Similar disturbances can occur in migraine. People or surrounding objects or parts of the patient's own body may appear to grow smaller or larger in "Alice in Wonderland" style. Lewis Carroll suffered from migraine, and it has been postulated that his migraine experiences may have inspired some of Alice's adventures. One patient of mine described her fingers feeling as long as telephone poles while her mouth felt as large as a cave with the teeth sticking up in it "like a row of tombstones."

Loss of concentration is usual at the peak of a migraine attack, and this may progress to a complete state of confusion in some patients. One patient of mine left her child alone in the bath and was found running down the street outside her house. A few patients may become very sleepy and hard to awaken while the attack lasts. Others may experience hallucinations like a series of nightmares.

Instead of the weakness of one side, which has been called hemiplegic migraine, the occasional patient may notice involuntary movements of one arm and leg. In one patient of mine the movements were very similar to those seen in rheumatic chorea ("St. Vitus's dance").

Most patients cannot tolerate light when the headache becomes severe and prefer to lie in a darkened room. All the senses may become acute, so that they cannot bear noises or smells, even those which may normally be pleasant. The scalp is usually tender during the headache and may remain sensitive for a day or so afterward. Even combing or brushing the hair may require a delicate touch.

Fluid is usually retained in the body before and during the migraine attack so that the hands and feet may become swollen, the face puffy, and the abdomen distended. Many comment on passing large amounts of urine as the headache subsides and the excess bodily fluid is excreted. Unfortunately, the use of drugs which help to rid the body of retained salt and water has not proved effective in preventing migraine in the past but, with the advent of more effective new agents, this approach may be worth re-exploring.

Nausea, which is almost universal, is not a reaction to the pain of migraine since it may precede the headache in some patients. The majority of patients vomit with severe attacks and some 20 percent pass several loose bowel movements during the headache. Many patients say that their headache starts to improve as soon as they vomit, and some deliberately make themselves sick because it helps to make their headache go away.

In addition to the pallor, pulsation of scalp arteries,

and prominent veins that have been mentioned, the eyes may become bloodshot and some patients have noticed "blood spots" in the eye or bruising elsewhere in the face. Tissot in 1834 commented, "The eye on the affected side is sometimes suffused. Sometimes it is even very red during the attack." He reported one lady in whom "it was no uncommon occurrence with her in the severer seizures for the violence of the spasm to occasion an extraversation of blood, rendering the skin of the forehead, eyelids, and even the cheeks black and blue."

Chills and cold sweats may accompany some headaches although a fever is rare. However, Dr. Oliver Sachs in his book on migraine reported that one of his patients developed a fever of 103.5°F in such attacks.

THE NATURE OF THE HEADACHE

The headache may start with a dull pain in the upper part of the neck on one side and spread forward to involve the whole head. It may remain localized to the forehead or one temple or may radiate backward from these regions until one-half of the head or the entire head is aching. The aching usually spreads down to the neck but rarely to the shoulders and upper arms.

Occasionally, the pain affects the face below the eye rather than the head. In this case, the pain spreads to the cheek, nostril, ear, and jaw. The nostril may be blocked on the painful side. This variation of migraine is known as "lower-half headache" or "facial migraine."

The frequency of migraine attacks varies from once in a lifetime to several each year, several each week, or even daily. The greater the frequency of the attacks, the more significant is the part which psychological factors play and the more important it becomes to seek sources of anxiety or depression in the sufferer's personal background. Other causes of increasing frequency of migraine include contraceptive pills and high blood pressure.

The headache may last a few hours only, disappearing with rest or sleep, or may persist for a day or several days. After the acute ache disappears, a tense bruised tender feeling may persist in the muscles for hours or days.

The pain may be present when waking up in the morning or may even awaken the patient at 3:00 or 4:00 A.M. If it comes on during the day, it may be preceded by a dull ache or by the more spectacular visual or other cerebral symptoms which were discussed earlier.

In the early stages the headache is commonly throbbing, meaning that it becomes worse with each beat of the pulse. It may then be transmuted into a constant pain, which can become very severe unless effective treatment is used early.

THE NATURAL HISTORY OF MIGRAINE

It is quite common for migraine to take different forms at different ages. The young child may be subject to recurrent vomiting attacks with little or no accompanying headache. At the age of six or seven, the headache usually becomes a more conspicuous feature. After puberty, the headache may be preceded by patchy loss of vision and flashes of light in front of the eyes or other neurological symptoms. As time goes on, vomiting subsides so that the middle-aged patient may experience only loss of appetite or mild nausea with the headache. After menopause the headaches usually become less frequent and may disappear altogether. In some patients the cerebral symptoms may persist in isolation as a "migraine equivalent." At any age there may be periods of freedom from headache lasting for years. These often cannot be ascribed to any particular change in personality or environment. Relief from migraine in the later years of life cannot be promised. Doctors C. W. M. Whitty and J. M. Hockaday in Oxford found that about half of the patients they checked up on still complained of headaches in their sixties. I have looked after one patient in her eighties who is still plagued by frequent and severe migraine.

INTERFERENCE WITH SCHOOL AND WORK

Professor Bo Bille of Uppsala, Sweden, reported that girls with migraine lost an average of fifty hours from school each term compared with an average of twenty-seven hours for girls who were not subject to headache. There was no difference between migrainous and non-migrainous boys. The impact of migraine is probably a lot greater than this in the school years. Concentration may be impaired and motivation may flag, so that the net loss may be more serious than appears from the statistics. In addition, children may miss out on many of the minor but important joys of childhood.

Those adults most severely afflicted by migraine cannot carry out any useful work. At the other end of the scale, patients who rarely experience migraine, or who have attacks only on weekends (see Chapter 9), or whose headache respond promptly to treatment lose no time at all. Doctors K. M. Gammie and W. E. Waters found that 17 percent of all workers attending the medical clinic in an English factory did so on account of headache. Doctor Waters also collaborated with a London general practitioner, Dr. G. J. R. Clarke. Their article concluded:

There is very little information on the duration of sickness absence due to headaches. The figures produced
by sickness benefit statistics include only absences of
more than three days and for which sickness benefit is
claimed. In 1968/9 there were 295,000 man days (and
167,000 woman days) recorded as lost through migraine
in Britain (Office of Health Economics, 1972). From the
results of the present survey the total amount from all
headaches is many times this number although further
studies will be required to see if the present figures are
typical of the time lost from headaches in the country
as a whole.

HOW COMMON IS MIGRAINE?

It has always been difficult to assess the number of patients in a community who suffer from migraine. Some
may have had only one or two attacks in their lives and
may not consider this worth mentioning in any survey.
On the other hand, there are those whose headaches
are not really migrainous, but an inaccurate description
may lead to their being classified as migraine. Estimates
of the incidence in different surveys have varied from
3 percent to 9 percent of the population.

It is probably more helpful to consider each age
group separately. Professor Bille studied nine thousand
Swedish children and found that 1 percent suffered
from migraine at the age of six years and that the proportion increased with age until 4 percent of boys and
5 to 6 percent of girls were affected by the age of twelve
years. Professor Dalsgaard-Nielsen in Denmark found a
slightly higher incidence at each age and noted that
there was a marked sex difference in the susceptibility
to migraine from the age of puberty onward. During
the reproductive period of life from puberty until the
forties, some 19 percent of women were liable to mi-

graine, while the figures for males remained about half that for females. These statistics are almost identical with those of Doctors W. E. Waters and P. J. O'Connor who conducted a similar survey in Wales. This accounts for the female preponderance among patients thronging doctors' offices with the problem of migraine. About 70 percent of the patients are women.

Not all patients with migraine consult a doctor. Waters found that about half the people subject to migraine had never consulted a doctor about their headaches.

CONCLUSION

Migraine is a common disorder which interferes with normal life and destroys much of the pleasure in life when it is severe and recurs frequently. It is essentially an episodic disorder in which blood is shunted away from the cerebral cortex and the scalp. As a result, the unfortunate sufferer may undergo a wide variety of symptoms. While the smaller vessels are constricted, the arteries dilate, giving rise to a headache that is commonly one-sided. The headache is usually accompanied by nausea, vomiting, and sensitivity to light. The varied manifestations of migraine can be explained in terms of disordered control of blood vessels which overreact in response to emotional, physical, and chemical stimuli.

9

The Causes of Migraine

It is not possible at the moment to give a short simple answer to the question "What is the cause of migraine?" We can, however, identify a chain of events. It starts with various trigger factors, described later, and ends with changes in the dimensions of the blood vessels. We know that the person who suffers from migraine has blood vessels which are particularly sensitive to any stimulus such as a head injury or alteration in the immediate environment of the vessels. Such a change might be brought about by levels of chemical messengers in the blood stream. We know that the end result is a constriction of small vessels and a swelling of large vessels so that blood is shunted away from the periphery to flow more rapidly from arteries to veins without serving its purpose of bringing oxygen to the peripheral areas of the brain and scalp. We do not fully understand the intermediate steps which play the part of the middlemen in the transaction.

What sort of person gets migraine? The fact that women are more liable to migraine than men in the ratio of about three to one has already been mentioned. The observation that about one-quarter of all patients date the onset of their migraine to childhood and that a family history of the disorder is present in more than half is also important. For comparison, patients with tension headaches or other adults who are not prone to headaches have a family history of migraine in less than one-fifth of cases, a highly significant difference. Moreover, Professor Bille in Sweden found that 78 percent of migrainous children had a positive family history in contrast to 18 percent of the control group.

PERSONALITY AND INTELLIGENCE

In the past, migraine patients have received some consolation from the assurance that the disorder strikes only those who are intelligent and sensitive. While the second part of this proposition may be true, the evidence unfortunately does not support the idea that migraine sufferers are brighter than average. Bille did not find any difference in the school marks achieved by migrainous and nonmigrainous groups of children, and he could not detect any indications of greater ambition in the migrainous children.

The person susceptible to migraine is said to be tense, meticulous, and obsessional by nature. In a group of five hundred patients studied by Dr. George Selby and myself, 23 percent were found to be unduly tidy and house-proud and had the habit of double-checking their actions. Another 22 percent were overactive, restless, and tense individuals who found it very difficult to relax. Definite symptoms of anxiety were present in another 13 percent who experienced difficulty in sleeping, tremor of the hands, a tendency to take deep, sighing breaths, and feelings of depression.

To come to any valid conclusions, it is necessary to compare a control group of similar age, sex, and social background who are not subject to migraine. Bille found that migrainous children were significantly more anxious, tense, sensitive, and vulnerable to frustration than the control children. In addition, the migraine-prone children were more tidy and less strong than their peers. Doctors Rita Henryk-Gutt and W. Linford Rees of St. Bartholomew's Hospital, London, studied fifty men and fifty women from the Civil Service. They compared them with matched controls, who suffered from other forms of headache, and with another group who were not prone to any kind of headache. They found that migraine sufferers had not been exposed to more stress than the other groups but that they reacted more to all forms of stress. They could not confirm previous suggestions that they were more obsessional or ambitious. More than half the episodes of migraine were attributed to some obviously stressful event.

EPILEPSY AND ALLERGY

An analogy has often been drawn between epilepsy and migraine because both often appear suddenly in those who are otherwise well, and both may recur at fairly regular intervals. To assess whether epilepsy was more common in migraine subjects, Dr. Michael Anthony and I compared a group of five hundred patients who were subject to typical migraine attacks with one hundred patients who had only tension headaches. There was no difference between the two groups in their liability to epilepsy or in any family history of epilepsy. Bille came to identical conclusions in his study of migrainous children.

A similar analysis has been made of adults and children to see whether allergic disorders (asthma, hay fever, hives, and eczema) were more common in patients who suffered from migraine. The frequency of allergy was found to be no greater than that in the populations with which they were compared. This does not mean that an allergic attack may not occasionally trigger migraine or that a severe migraine headache may not occasionally precipitate an epileptic attack in someone *who is already predisposed to epilepsy from some other cause.* This is quite a different matter from trying to link these disorders to a common underlying cause, for which there is no evidence whatever.

TRIGGER FACTORS

Many patients can identify specific circumstances which commonly lead to migraine headache. These are not necessarily *causes* of migraine but may set in motion the mysterious machinery which results in an episode of migraine. Certainly the most direct of these triggers is a blow to the head.

Blows to the head (footballer's migraine)
It has been suspected for a long time that a severe head injury may be responsible for the onset of migraine, particularly if scalp vessels have been damaged by lacerations at the time of injury. It has not been realized that a blow to the head may lead to the onset of migrainous symptoms within a few minutes. Professor W. B. Matthews of Oxford University has recently described a group of young male patients whose blurring of vision followed within two minutes after being hit on the head by a football or being punched in a boxing match. The attacks progressed to typical migraine headache with vomiting. Curiously enough, none was subject to headache on either occasion. Doctors David Haas and Robert Sovner in Syracuse, New York, described migrainous symptoms, numbness and weakness of one side of the body, and speech difficulty after mild head injuries in children. These symptoms were followed by sick headaches in most. There was a family tendency, two children and one adult in one family having had this experience and a father and son in another. The attacks started twenty minutes or more

after injuries that were quite minor, such as falling off
a couch, bumping heads together while playing, and
falling on ice.

These observations are important for two reasons.
First, anxiety may be allayed when one realizes that
some frightening symptoms after a blow to the head
may be migrainous and do not necessarily indicate serious damage to the brain. Second, any explanation of
migraine must explain the onset of symptoms within
minutes after the blow. Doctors Haas and Sovner believe that arteries at the base of the brain may go into
spasm when the head is suddenly jarred by the injury.
Perhaps the blow may also initiate some of the chemical changes which we shall consider later.

Changes in barometric pressure

Classic migraine has been reported by airplane crews
at a high altitude and, more commonly, five to thirty
minutes after descent. It has also been reported after
recovery from simulated altitudes of thirty to thirty-
eight thousand feet in a low-pressure chamber. It tends
to occur repeatedly in certain individuals, particularly
those who have previously suffered from migraine, and
not at all in others. Headache is also a common symptom of "acute mountain sickness" when healthy people
remain at a simulated altitude of fourteen to fifteen
thousand feet for several hours. It is caused by swelling
of the scalp arteries and is relieved by pressure on these
vessels or by drugs which cause the arteries to constrict.

Decompression after simulated diving to depths of
66 to 135 feet below sea level in a high-pressure (hyperbaric) chamber has also been known to precipitate migraine. Four out of thirty individuals who were exposed
weekly to such pressure changes experienced the sensation of flashing lights, "heat waves," or rainbows in

front of their eyes with blurring of vision ten to ninety minutes after decompression, in most cases followed later by headache. The visual disturbances disappeared promptly with oxygen therapy, but the headache still followed in three out of four subjects. All four were subject to migraine at other times, but the induced attacks differed from the spontaneous attacks, being milder in some and more severe in others.

The arteries of the scalp and brain appear to be very sensitive to the pressure of oxygen in the blood and particularly to any sudden change in its level.

Weather
Many patients believe that sudden changes in the weather, particularly thunderstorms, may be responsible for migraine. Although the drop in barometric pressure is not nearly as dramatic as that in compression chambers, the possibility that it plays some part in triggering migraine, possibly by increasing nervous tension, cannot be denied. Professor F. G. Sulman and his colleagues have studied the effect of a hot, dry wind, known as the Sharav, in Israel. They point out that cool winds like the French Mistral or Canadian Chinook do not usually cause headache but that "hot winds of ill repute" are notorious for causing irritability, depression, and headache. They list the Santa Ana of southern California, Arizona desert winds, the Argentine Zonda, the Sirocco of the Mediterranean, the Maltese Xlokk, the Chamsin of Arab countries, the Sharav of the Old Testament, the Foehn of Switzerland, southern Germany, and Austria, and the North Winds of Melbourne. They found that a "weather front" with increased ionization of the air (electrical changes which may cause lightning) arrived one to two days before the hot, dry wind and considered that this might be responsible for

the symptoms. Of two hundred patients who developed symptoms with the Sharav, eighty excreted excessive amounts of serotonin (a substance which is thought to play a part in causing migraine). Migraine was prevented in seventy of these cases by the use of pills which counteracted the effect of serotonin.

Stress (emotions, glare, noise)

Some degree of stress must be associated with receiving a blow on the head or being locked in a decompression chamber. One patient of mine regularly had a migraine headache the day after he had his hair cut. It would be taking an extreme view to classify a haircut as a head injury, Samson notwithstanding. Perhaps this may be regarded as a form of stress. Emotional stress can certainly provoke a migraine headache. Several of my patients have mentioned that the distortion of vision which heralds an attack started within minutes of an emotional shock. In their survey of migraine patients Doctors Henryk-Gutt and Rees found that about half their patients attributed the onset of attacks to some obviously stressful event.

Other factors such as noise, glare, smells, or unpleasant weather conditions, like hot, dry winds, can induce nervous tension and evoke an attack of migraine. Some 50 percent of patients blame the glare from driving a car into the sun or watching movies or television. Sensitivity to noise was described by the French physician Labarraque in 1837 in the following terms:

> We all know that it is not everyone who can, with impunity, do himself the pleasure of assisting at certain theatrical representations where the glory of France is daily celebrated with noise and smoke. And how many good citizens are there not, tried patriots, whom the

threatening of a migraine, infallibly brought on by the unaccustomed din of drums and military music, forcibly hinders from taking part in our civic fêtes, and joining their companies on grand review days.

Relaxation after stress (weekend headache)

When headaches appear only on weekends, there is no need necessarily to blame the domestic situation. It is probable that during prolonged periods of stress, the scalp vessels are constricted by the nervous system or by chemicals in the blood stream such as serotonin and norepinephrine. When the working week ends and the subject is able to relax at last, the vessels tend to dilate and cause migraine headache. Doctor Arnold P. Friedman in his essay "The Headache in History, Literature and Legend" quotes from a letter by Sigmund Freud who wrote, "My health has been excellent—regulated by a slight migraine on Sundays."

Sleeping in on Saturday or Sunday mornings may also be a factor causing weekend headache, possibly because the depth of respiration decreases during some phases of sleep, permitting the accumulation of carbon dioxide in the blood. Carbon dioxide is known to be a potent dilator of intracranial blood vessels, so an excessive amount in the blood could cause headache.

Just as relaxation may induce headache, a sudden emotion may cure it. Doctor Friedman also quotes an example of this. Ulysses S. Grant, general of the Union armies in the Civil War, was "suffering very severely from a sick headache" and spent the night bathing his feet in hot water and mustard and putting mustard plasters on his wrists and neck. The next day he received a letter from Robert E. Lee, the Confederate general, announcing that he was willing to surrender. Grant wrote in his journal, "I was still suffering from the

sick headache: but the instant I saw the contents of the
note I was cured." He later commented, "The pain in
my head seemed to leave me the moment I got Lee's
letter." The nineteenth-century French physician
Labarraque described the prevention of an attack by a
sudden shock. A thirty-five-year-old woman suffered
from migraine every eight to ten days. "One day when
she felt an attack coming on, going to look at her face
in the glass, her cap caught fire and burnt her forehead.
The expected seizure never came on, and furthermore,
she had no return for some years."

Sleep

A jailer in Shakespeare's *Cymbeline* says, "Indeed,
sir, he that sleeps feels not the toothache." Unfortunately, sir and madame, he that sleeps does feel the
headache. Indeed it is not uncommon for a person to be
awakened by a headache in the small hours of the
morning, or for one to be present when he or she awakens at his usual time. Doctors Dexter and Weitzman in
Dr. Friedman's department at the Montefiore Hospital
in New York studied a number of patients who were
plagued with nocturnal headache by recording their
brain waves, the electrical activity of the brain, while
they slept. This was done by attaching electrodes to the
scalp, and the changes in electrical activity were written out as an electroencephalogram (EEG). It is well
known that the EEG pattern alters during the various
stages of sleep. At intervals throughout the night, sleep
lightens. As this happens, the brain waves indicate partial arousal and the eyes move from side to side. This is
known as the rapid eye movement (REM) phase of
sleep. At the onset of REM sleep, all sorts of activity
may happen, such as dreams, nocturnal emissions, and
even bed-wetting. All the nocturnal headaches ob-

served were related to the REM phase of sleep. It is interesting to note that dreams and headache may become intermingled. Liveing quoted an example: "Dr. Airy says his attacks sometimes occur in the night, and that he has had an indistinct consciousness of having experienced the visual phenomena in his sleep, mixed up with his dreams, and he awakes in the second, or headache stage." When the cycle of sleeping and waking is altered in phase (for example by air travel), headaches also change in timing, but maintain their relation to the REM phase of sleep. Doctor John Graham of Boston told me that a patient of his who often flew from the east to Los Angeles continued to have his headaches on eastern standard time for several days before he adjusted his sleep (and headache) rhythm to local time. Whether REM sleep and its associated headache is related to changes in brain chemistry, or to the accumulation of carbon dioxide in the blood stream, or to other factors is at present unknown.

Foods

Headaches have long been attributed to disturbances of digestion and to the flow of bile, one of the digestive juices. The vomiting attacks of childhood, often migrainous in origin, are still referred to as "bilious attacks." The Roman physician Galen commented almost two thousand years ago, "How constantly do we see the head attacked with pain when yellow bile is contained in the stomach: as also the pain forthwith ceasing when the bile has been vomited."

The belief that migraine may be triggered by taking certain kinds of foods is of equally long standing. Doctor John Fothergill, a London physician, wrote in 1778: "It is most clear that the headache proceeds from the stomach, not the reverse." He blamed certain foods, particularly "melted butter, fat meats, spices, meat pies, hot buttered toast, and malt liquors when strong and hoppy." Fothergill went on to add, "From many incontestible proofs that butter in considerable quantity is injurious, it is less used in many families. Nothing more speedily and effectively gives the sick-headache, and sometimes within a few hours."

Occasionally migraine may be preceded by an intense desire to eat a certain type of food, particularly sweet things, including chocolate. Liveing told of a patient who could "devour a whole tin of biscuits without being satisfied" immediately before her migraine headache.

When Dr. George Selby and I analyzed the case histories of five hundred migraine patients, we found that 25 percent attributed the onset on occasions to eating certain foods (compared with 67 percent who blamed emotional disturbances and 47 percent who mentioned glare). Fats, fried foods, chocolates, and oranges were most often cited, but tomatoes, pineapples, and onions were also occasionally mentioned. Before becoming carried away with the food-sensitivity hypothesis, one would do well to consider some experiments carried out by the late Harold G. Wolff at New York Hospital. "With the administration of chocolate disguised in capsules for those allegedly sensitive to chocolate, or milk given through a stomach tube to those who were said to be sensitive to milk, the results did not confirm the earlier work. No headache ensued." A recent study from The London Hospital of twenty-five patients who claimed that their headaches were invariably brought on by eating chocolate or any cocoa products could not find any relationship. In eighty trials, only thirteen headaches followed the taking of chocolate, while eight came on after eating a substance which had been made to look like chocolate.

In our own clinic, thirty-four migrainous patients were skin-tested for food and other allergies. Twenty-three patients who gave positive reactions avoided the appropriate allergens for several months without reduction in the frequency of attacks. Ten patients were placed on low-fat diets for up to six months, but again the pattern of attacks remained unaltered. It is thus unlikely that any change in diet will make a substantial difference to the migraine patient. There is certainly no need for anyone who is subject to migraine to avoid fatty foods, chocolate, oranges, or other food unless he or she has strong personal reasons for doing so.

The eating of cheese has recently come into prominence because Dr. E. Hanington and her colleagues in London found that tyramine, which is present in cheese, could produce a migraine headache in susceptible patients whereas lactose given in identical capsules rarely did. However, a recent repetition of this experiment by another group in London found that headache followed the taking of the same amount of tyramine no more frequently than the inactive substance with which tyramine was compared. This subject therefore remains *sub judice* at the moment.

Missing meals

While it is doubtful that foods trigger migraine, there is little question that missing meals may cause headache in some people, probably by lowering the blood sugar level. Doctor J. N. Blau and Professor J. N. Cumings of The National Hospital for Nervous Diseases in London found that six out of twelve migrainous subjects who did not eat for nineteen hours developed a migraine headache. A follow-up of this study by Dr. Blau and Dr.

D. A. Pyke involved the investigation of thirty-six patients with both migraine and diabetes. Six patients noted that missing a meal provoked migraine headache, and another four were subject to headaches at night, when their blood sugar fell as a result of insulin treatment. The patients could differentiate between the onset of migraine and the generalized headache which usually accompanied a severe drop in the blood sugar level after insulin, and some felt that they could prevent the development of migraine by eating as soon as they felt the first symptoms. The effect of lowering blood sugar by giving insulin to nondiabetic migraine patients is less effective. Doctor John Pearce of Hull, England, found that only two out of twenty responded with a headache.

Alcohol
Wine is mentioned as a precipitant of migraine in the days of the Roman Empire. Cornelius Celsus, a friend of the emperor Tiberius, wrote in about A.D. 30 of a headache "sometimes afflicting the whole head, at other times a part of it," contracted by drinking wine and recurring throughout life. Edward Liveing in 1873 commented, "Some few individuals cannot tolerate any kind of beer or wine." He quoted a case: "One gentleman, a most intelligent member of our profession . . . told me that for twenty years or more he could never take the smallest quantity of wine (and he mentioned the sacramental wine as an instance) . . . without infallibly producing a headache." In general, Liveing considered "wine, especially if taken in larger quantity, or of a different quality from that to which the patient is accustomed, or if several kinds are taken, will often occasion an attack; but this is not the case when the same kind is taken daily with moderation and

regularity; and with many patients it is very beneficial."
In fact, he states that "a full dose of Brandy or other
alcoholic stimulant, if taken sufficiently early, will occasionally disperse an incipient seizure [of migraine]."

I have not encountered any patient who could prevent an attack by taking alcohol in any form. In fact, it
is usually a useful point in distinguishing a vascular
headache, such as migraine, from tension headache.
Tension headache is often relieved by alcohol; vascular
headaches are almost invariably made worse. The reason for this is that alcohol is a dilator of blood vessels and
that the pain of migraine arises from vessels which are
already dilated.

A further complication is that certain wines, particularly red wines, contain tyramine and histamine.
These have a potent dilator effect in addition to that
of alcohol and are therefore well equipped to spring
the migraine trap. I have seen many patients, including neurologists and other physicians, who are con-
vinced that their migraines follow the drinking of
red wines but who may enjoy white wines without
any problem. One interesting point is that a trigger
such as red wine may not be effective immediately
after a spontaneous headache or for some days afterward until the vessels regain their sensitivity. It is as
though the vessels are exhausted after an attack and
enter a refractory period during which they will not
respond, however great the provocation.

Exercise
A number of patients develop migraine after extreme exertion like playing a hard game of tennis. Such
headaches may usually be prevented by taking suitable
medication, such as ergotamine tartrate or methysergide, before the exercise starts. These medications pre-

vent painful swelling of the scalp arteries and are discussed later in the treatment of migraine.

Hormonal changes

The character of migraine frequently undergoes a transformation at puberty. The more dramatic symptoms of visual and sensory disturbance often appear then for the first time, and the headaches may become more intense than ever before. In pubescent girls, the incidence of migraine increases until twice as many girls are affected as boys. In some 60 percent of female patients, headaches occur before or during menstruation. In the last six months of pregnancy, the majority obtain some relief, only to have the headache attacks recur shortly after the delivery of their baby. Doctor Michael Anthony and I studied 120 women who had undergone 252 pregnancies and found that relief during pregnancy was more common in those women whose migraine had previously been associated with their menstrual periods (64 percent) than in those in whom it had not (48 percent). A few women notice the onset of migraine for the first time during pregnancy, but these are in the minority.

Doctor Brian Somerville in my division at The Prince Henry Hospital, Sydney, has studied levels of female hormones in the blood throughout the menstrual cycle in a number of migrainous women. The headache always started while the levels of estrogen and progesterone were falling before the onset of menstruation. Somerville found that injections of progesterone to maintain a high level in the blood did not prevent the onset of migraine, but that injections of estrogen would delay the headache until the level in the blood finally dropped. We may conclude that the fall of the level of estrogen in some way triggers off migraine.

Menstruation comes about when the constriction of the small blood vessels which supply the soft inner lining of the uterus causes the superficial layers to slough off and discharge in the menstrual flow. There is some evidence that members of a group of substances called the prostaglandins are responsible for this constriction of vessels in the womb, and it is also known that other members of this group can cause migraine if injected into the blood stream of people who have never had a migraine attack before in their lives. It is tempting to guess that the lowering of the female hormone estradiol in the blood releases prostaglandins. These may set in train the vascular changes of menstruation and, as a side effect in some unfortunate individuals, the vascular changes which result in migraine.

Oral contraceptives contain differing combinations of synthetic estrogens and progesterones which prevent ovulation. They do not really simulate the changes of pregnancy because the blood level is permitted to fall away at monthly intervals to allow menstruation to take place. A few patients notice an improvement in their migraine when they start taking one form or other of "the pill," but in most patients the frequency and intensity of headaches increase, and some notice additional minor vascular headaches. Almost all patients continue to have a migraine attack before their periods. Those whose migraine is worsened by oral contraceptives must decide whether or not to continue taking them, which would mean adding daily medication to diminish their sensitivity to migraine (like driving a car with the accelerator and the brake being applied together). Alternatively, they can stop the pill and run the risk of an unwanted pregnancy. In one group of patients, the policy of our clinic is very clear. All those who have severe intracranial symptoms with their attacks—speech difficulty, pins and needles or weakness down one side of the body, or loss of vision—are advised in the strongest terms to stop taking oral contraceptives. In a number of instances, sufferers from this form of migraine have sustained a permanent disability resembling a stroke when they have continued to take the pill regularly. In ordinary forms of migraine, "common migraine," the choice is left to the patient.

Migraine without any precipitating factors

While all of the situations and circumstances described above may trigger migraine attacks, many patients go on having their attacks without relation to any external pressures.

Doctor Arnold P. Friedman told of one of his patients who "has an occupation that takes him through the world from the Himalayas in Tibet to Somaliland, indeed from the highest altitudes to the lowest, from the wettest to the driest—experiencing climatic, food and culture changes. But his migraine remains, for he carries his personal environment with him."

10

The Mechanism of Migraine

WHAT CAUSES THE HEADACHE?

There is no doubt that the pain of migraine arises from dilated blood vessels. The large arteries and possibly also the large veins in the scalp are primarily responsible, but the arteries inside the skull contribute in some patients, particularly those who feel the pain deeply behind one eye. Patients of mine have commented that they can relieve pain in the temples or forehead by pressing on the temporal artery (felt as a pulse just in front of the ear, shown in Figure 2) but that pain persists behind the eye. The relief of pain by pressure on the arteries of the scalp was noted by Möllendorf in the mid-nineteenth century: "If the common carotid artery be forcibly compressed on the painful side . . . so that the pulse in the temporal artery begins to fail, the headache vanishes as if by magic."

Local pressure also relieves the pain. Queen Mary Tudor was afflicted by migraine during her coronation. Doctor Macdonald Critchley quoted from her biography: "Mary rode in an open litter, clad in splendid blue velvet, with a jewelled diadem so heavy that its weight on the usual headache—she was having one of her bad days—was sheer agony, so that for part of the way she tried to ease the blind pain by resting her head on her hand."

Anything which diminishes the flow in the affected arteries reduces the pain. In 1796, Erasmus Darwin, the grandfather of the great Charles Darwin, suggested a trial of centrifugal force which, as he quaintly intimated, "cannot be done in private practice, and which I therefore recommend to some hospital physician." He speculated, "What might be the consequence of whirling a person with his head next to centre of motion, so as to force the blood from the brain into the other parts of the body? Would a circulating bed remove any kind of headache?" This challenge was taken up by Dr. Harold G. Wolff 150 years later, using a man-carrying centrifuge. He found that rotating a patient with the head centrally placed and the feet outward completely eliminated migraine headache in four patients when they were exposed to a force equivalent to twice that of gravity. Headaches caused by hunger and concussion were also relieved by centrifuging, showing that they too resulted from dilatation of blood vessels.

Wolff continued his observations by studying the effects of stimulating exposed scalp arteries of volunteers who remained conscious and described their sensations. When an artery was distended by stretching its wall with a clamp placed inside the vessel, the subject felt pain in the area over the artery. Threads were then attached to the wall of the artery and pulled rhythmically so that a throb of pain was felt every time the artery was widened. This procedure was then carried out at two points on the temporal artery, and the throbbing pain extended from in front of the ear to the forehead and the subject started to feel nauseated. This experiment simulated closely the pain of migraine, and the stoic subjects are to be congratulated if not envied for their contribution to scientific knowledge.

If dilatation of the blood vessels causes headache, why do we not get one every time we take a hot bath or play a game of tennis? Most people don't. After exercise or other forms of body heating, the arteries are certainly distended. We can feel their increased pulsation by placing our fingers in front of each ear. The face is flushed and veins on the forehead stand out, showing that blood is flowing freely through the skin and vessels underlying it into the draining veins. Blood does not bank up in the arteries. However, in migraine the face is usually pale. Blood flow is bypassing the skin, but it is not known whether or not the pressure is increased in the dilated scalp arteries. We do know that these arteries are more sensitive to pain than usual, probably because of the accumulation of chemical substances around them. Wolff found a substance resembling bradykinin around the scalp arteries during migraine headache. Professor Federigo Sicuteri of Florence has shown that the combination of bradykinin and serotonin will produce pain in blood vessels, and we know that serotonin is released from its body stores during migraine attacks. We thus have a simple hypothesis: The arteries of migraine are painful when dilated because they are sensitized by bradykinin and serotonin.

WHAT CAUSES THE OTHER SYMPTOMS OF MIGRAINE?

Before the flow increases in the arteries of the brain and scalp, the small branches of arteries which supply the cerebral cortex are constricted. Intracranial pressure is low when the blood supply to the brain is diminished and increases as the blood flow increases. In 1935, Goltman described the strange fluctuations in size of the brain during migraine attacks in a woman who had a bone defect in her skull. The pressure inside the skull could be judged by whether the scalp was bulging over the bone defect or was sunken inward. Goltman noted, "Immediately before the onset of the headache attack her face appeared blanched, at which time there was a definite depression at the site of the bone defect." Then as the headache developed, "the skull depression began to fill up, and ultimately the intracranial contents protruded, assuming the appearance of a tumour. When it thus became a bulging mass it was not tender and did not pulsate on palpation. The patient then began to vomit. The pallor of the face gave way to a flush. After twelve to seventy-three hours the headache subsided and the intracranial contents resumed their former relation to the bone defect."

More specific information has come from X rays of the blood vessels taken during migraine and from studies of blood flow using radioactive isotopes. It is possible to obtain clear pictures of the arteries supplying the brain by injecting them with a material which does not transmit X rays, so that the whole arterial tree can be seen in silhouette. Such X rays (called arteriograms or angiograms) taken during the early phase of migraine, while visual and other sensory disturbances are in progress, have shown that the large arteries are usually normal in appearance. This suggests that it is only the smaller branches, not seen in the arteriogram, that constrict in this phase.

The electroencephalogram (EEG), which records the electrical "brain waves," shows an abnormal pattern in the area of the brain where the small vessels are constricted, depriving that area of blood. There seems to be little doubt that such constriction takes place. When radioactive xenon gas is inhaled or injected into the arteries, the passage of blood through different parts of the brain may be measured accurately by a Geiger counter placed on the head. These techniques have shown that blood flow is reduced by 50 percent in the parts of the brain which are giving rise to symptoms, showing that blood is shunted away from the cortex at that time. When cerebral symptoms disappear and headache follows, the blood flow *increases* up to 50 percent. Cerebral arteries must therefore dilate during the headache phase, as well as the scalp arteries which can be observed directly.

One facet that has not been explained is the slow spread of sensory disturbances in some patients. Zigzags of light may appear in one part of the visual field and slowly move across the field, leaving a patchy or complete loss of vision behind them. Doctor K. S. Lashley, a distinguished Harvard psychologist who was subject to this sort of visual hallucination, retained his spirit of scientific enquiry despite the advancing migrainous eclipse and sat in front of a dark screen on many occasions meticulously plotting the extent of his field of vision by sticking pins into the screen to mark its outer limits. As the outskirts of his vision shrank he constructed a series of contour lines on the screen to help him later determine the rate at which his sight had decreased. He calculated that the cortex of his brain must have been thrown out of action by some process which moved across its surface at the speed of three millimeters each minute.

Now it so happens that there is a process well known to physiologists which executes a slow march across the cortex at precisely three millimeters per minute, called "spreading depression," caused by a change in the membrane of nerve cells. Moreover, it is preceded by a constriction of small vessels and is followed by their dilatation. It seems highly probable that this process underlies the gradual onset of the cerebral symptoms which many patients experience, the slow growth of numbness over one side of the body, the plucking out one by one of the words required for coherent speech, and the progressive suffocation of the intellect which is a transient but disturbing part of the migraine syndrome in some patients.

Why should the visual symptoms sometimes comprise flashes or pinpoints of light and sometimes shimmering or jittering zigzags of color? Recent experimental work has given some insight into this problem.

Doctors D. H. Hubel and T. N. Wiesel of Boston have shown that the part of the brain concerned with vision, the visual cortex, is arranged in sheets or columns of cells, each of which responds selectively to a bar of light held at a certain angle in front of the eye. As the angle of the bar is slowly rotated, one column of cells after another is thrown into activity. If we imagine the reverse of this process, any stimulation of a column of brain cells would cause a person to "see" a bar of light at a certain angle to the horizontal. If a wave of excitation crept over the visual cortex, the patient would see a succession of bars of light at different angles shimmering or jittering as column after column was stimulated. This is what happens in migraine. A wave of excitation sweeps over the cortex causing symptoms like zigzag lights in front of the eyes, followed by a period of depression of vision when the patient cannot see clearly.

If, on the other hand, the whole visual cortex is irritated at once by shunting blood away from the entire surface of the brain, the cells at the outer end of each column (farthest away from the source of blood supply) would fire off singly or in groups, giving the impression of stars or flashes of light rather than bars or zigzags. This is a common experience with some migraine patients. Doctors G. S. Brindley and B. S. Lewin stimulated the visual cortex of blind people by electrodes in an attempt to reproduce a pattern of vision which the patient can "see." The patients reported seeing fine points of white light like distant stars in the sky. We therefore have a plausible explanation for the visual symptoms of migraine, depending on whether the cortical function is impaired diffusely and simultaneously or progressively by a process spreading sideways over the surface.

What could be responsible for constriction of small vessels and the associated changes in cortical function? It is most likely to be a response peculiar to the blood vessels themselves, say in response to head injury, or occurring as a reaction to some chemical substance in the blood stream.

Why should patients with migraine wish to flee from the light and seek refuge in a darkened room? This aspect of migraine (megrim) was alluded to in a poem by Alexander Pope, who suffered from the disorder.

> And screen'd in shades from day's detested glare,
> She sighs for ever on her pensive bed,
> Pain at her side, and megrim at her head.

It was thought that dislike of light (photophobia) was caused by changes in the blood vessels in the white of the eye because these vessels commonly constrict in the early stages of an attack and dilate later on so that the eye appears bloodshot. Another theory involved irritation of the nerve supply to the eye from the pain of migraine. Neither of these explanations is completely satisfactory, for many patients also become acutely aware of smells and sounds. Smells that would be pleasing under normal circumstances may become an unbearable stench at the height of migraine headache, and background noise that customarily passes un-noticed may seem intolerable. There is surely a lower-ing of activity in the nervous connections which nor-mally modify perception from the special senses so that incoming information becomes magnified in migraine. Professor Federigo Sicuteri has recently postulated that this is caused by the loss of a chemical substance, seroto-nin, which is employed in transmission of nerve im-pulses between some nerve cells. He believes that the absence of serotonin also makes the person more aware of pain, so that ordinary background sensations give rise to a feeling of pain during migraine head-ache.

Nausea and vomiting are distressing symptoms of mi-graine at some time for most patients. Abdominal pain and diarrhea may also occur. It is quite common for people to remark on disturbances of appetite or bowel function immediately before the attack. Some may no-tice a greatly increased appetite or a craving for sweet things, even chocolate, which is often incriminated as a trigger factor for migraine (possibly for this reason). Others may lose their appetite. Another group com-plains of constipation. It seems that the whole gastro-intestinal tract is stilled before migraine starts—the calm before the storm. As the attack gathers momen-tum, waves of contraction are stirred up in the gastroin-testinal tract, reaching their climax in vomiting and sometimes diarrhea as well. Any explanation for this behavior cannot be based on the pain of migraine or the constriction of blood vessels supplying the vomiting center in the brain-stem. Nausea may precede the headache and brain-stem symptoms such as double vi-sion, slurred speech, loss of balance, and even giddiness may occur without nausea. The most acceptable hy-pothesis again implicates some chemical substance such as serotonin, that jack-of-all-trades, ubiquitous and potent. It is known that 95 percent of serotonin in the body is contained in the wall of the intestine and that the administration of serotonin increases intestinal activity. We also know that diarrhea is a major symptom of a carcinoid tumor, and carcinoid tumors manufacture large amounts of serotonin. It is possible that serotonin, which we know is released from its body stores during migraine, may be responsible for vomiting and diarrhea. This overactivity of the gastrointestinal tract may in turn release more serotonin from its hiding place in the intestinal wall.

What about the fluid retention which often accompanies migraine headache? Finger rings become tight, ankles swell noticeably, the face appears puffy—all these are signs of fluid retention. As the migraine attack wears off, large volumes of pale urine may be passed, thus eliminating excessive water from the body. At the risk of oversimplification, serotonin is also a possible cause of fluid retention because it can alter filtration in the kidney so that fluid is conserved in the body. Other hormones from the pituitary or adrenal glands can have the same effect.

NERVES OR CHEMICALS?

Emotion can induce migraine within minutes. A patient of mine was having a heated argument with a girlfriend about the rebellious attitude he had toward his father when he had been a teenager, a subject which had distressed him in later years. At the height of the argument his vision started to blur and soon he could see only the center of objects. This "tunnel vision" lasted for about ten minutes, after which his characteristic migraine headache developed. Some weeks later he was attending a cinema and found that the film dealt with the same problem of the father–son relationship which had always troubled him. The same sensation of distress swept over him. Within a few minutes his vision misted over, and tunnel vision was again followed by a headache.

What is the link between mind and body? Is the sequence of constriction and dilatation of blood vessels brought about by nerve pathways or by chemical messengers in the blood stream?

Certain reactions of the face and scalp are caused by the nerve fibers which form a network around blood vessels. These fibers are able to constrict the arteries of the scalp and brain but can dilate small vessels in the skin to produce blushing. Blushing is a good example of a vascular reaction produced by emotion through the nerve supply to the vessels. Since nerve pathways form the most direct link between mind and body, it is logical to think that they may be involved in migraine.

The vessels of the forehead are remarkably passive in their reactions except when they participate in blushing. When the external temperature suddenly drops or the body is cooled deliberately, vessels immediately constrict in the limbs so that the body conserves heat. The scalp vessels scarcely react at all. The forehead therefore continues to lose heat as the body cools. If the nerve supply to the scalp vessels is blocked by local anesthetic or severed, the pulsation of the arteries does not alter, indicating that the nerves are not normally exerting any controlling influence. Operations that have been devised to cut the nerve supply to blood vessels do not give any lasting benefit to patients with migraine. There is, therefore, no evidence that emotions can cause migraine through nerve pathways. There must be some chemical mediator, released at times of emotional stress, which can induce the vascular reactions responsible for migraine.

What are the known chemical agents which could be responsible? Bradykinin sensitizes blood vessels so that every pulsation of an artery is felt as a throbbing pain. It is a substance found wherever there is inflammation in the body and helps to cause the dilatation of blood vessels which makes the inflamed part red and swollen. It, or a substance very like it, has already been found around scalp arteries during migraine headache. If bradykinin is injected, it causes flushing and faintness but not headache, unless it is injected directly into the skin or muscle of the scalp. Then it causes local pain. It therefore appears that bradykinin could play a role in producing pain from the vessels but is not the chemical messenger we are seeking. It is interesting that aspirin will block the effect of bradykinin, which may be one way in which it helps to relieve pain.

Histamine is another substance which dilates blood vessels. It is the most important factor causing allergic reactions such as hives or hay fever, which are commonly treated by antihistamines. It is true that the level of histamine does slowly build up in the blood during migraine, but the process is so slow that it is almost certainly secondary to the attack and not the primary cause. There are some people whose migraine is consistently triggered by drinking red wines, which contain histamine, and the rare patient may complain of migraine regularly following an allergic reaction such as hay fever. In these cases histamine may act directly on the vessels or release other factors which do. However, the headache which has been induced by injecting histamine into human volunteers comes from the vessels inside the skull (intracranial vessels), and not from those in the scalp (extracranial vessels) which are mainly involved in migraine. Moreover, antihistamine agents have not proved very successful in preventing migraine.

The two most likely chemical substances at present appear to be serotonin and the prostaglandins. Serotonin was so named because it was found in the serum and gave "tone" to arteries by constricting them. Its chemical name is 5-hydroxytryptamine (5HT). It has a double-barreled action, tending to constrict large blood vessels and dilate small ones. This is the reverse of the situation in migraine, where the large arteries dilate and the small vessels constrict. We could, therefore, postulate that withdrawal of circulating serotonin could produce changes similar to those of migraine and giving serotonin to a patient might reverse or prevent the changes causing migraine. There is indeed evidence for both of these hypotheses. It has been shown that in most patients the level of serotonin in the blood drops sharply at the onset of migraine. A migraine attack can also be induced if the level is artificially lowered by drugs. Conversely, the intravenous injection of serotonin will reduce the pain of migraine or abolish it completely. Unfortunately, serotonin is not suitable for routine treatment because it causes unpleasant sensations of tightness in the chest, flushing, and pins and needles. Ergotamine tartrate is commonly given at the onset of migraine to shorten the attack. It is related chemically to serotonin and has a very similar effect on blood vessels. Some other preparations which are given regularly to prevent migraine, such as methysergide, have a tonic action on the scalp arteries similar to serotonin and may therefore be a substitute for it. Recently Professor Sicuteri has found that giving patients a precursor of serotonin by mouth reduces the frequency and severity of migraine attacks. Doctor Michael Anthony and I used a substance in treatment which stops the breakdown of serotonin in the body, and this also prevented migraine or reduced its severity. It looks, then, as though serotonin is on the side of the angels in the migraine story. Anything which increases blood serotonin helps. Anything which suddenly drops its level triggers off a headache. It seems that the rate of change in level is more important than the absolute level.

Interest has recently focused on a group of fatty acids called prostaglandins, of which one, prostaglandin E_1, looks the most promising. The prostaglandins are so called because they were first found in semen and were thought to come from the prostate gland. They were discovered in the search for the substance which makes the uterus contract when semen comes into contact with it. The prostaglandins that have this powerful effect on the uterus are in the "F" series, which also constricts blood vessels. It is thought that they are released before menstruation and constrict the blood vessels supplying the lining of the uterus. If members of the prostaglandin F series are released elsewhere in the body at this time, they could play a part in "menstrual migraine" by constricting the small vessels that supply the cerebral cortex.

The most interesting prostaglandin from our point of view is E_1, which dilates blood vessels. Some Scandinavian doctors infused prostaglandin E_1 into volunteers who had not been subject to migraine. All developed headache, abdominal pain, and nausea and became flushed and then pale. Most remarkable of all, two of the volunteers reported disturbances of vision described as "lightnings and other colored phenomena" followed by headache on one side of the head. Many studies are now in progress to see if any changes can be demonstrated in prostaglandins in the blood during a migraine attack.

We have considered a number of chemical substances which can induce changes in blood vessels of obvious relevance to the problem of migraine. They are sometimes called humoral agents after the four humors of classical medicine in Greek and Roman times. In the first chapter, a quotation from Paul of Aegina, written in A.D. 600, stated that headache is sometimes caused by a "redundance of humors." These words may prove to be a prophecy fulfilled in the twentieth century.

A COMPOSITE PICTURE

Let us look at the picture as a whole. On the one hand, we have a host of known trigger factors. On the other hand, we have an inherited sensitivity of blood vessels. In between, we have one or more steps involving circulating chemical agents.

Why should migraine affect only one side of the head in many people? Sometimes it may affect just one blood vessel predominantly. The headache may appear habitually on one side of the forehead, one temple, or one-half of the back of the head with tenderness over the upper part of the neck on that side. In these instances the major disturbance is clearly in the frontal, temporal, or occipital arteries which supply those areas of the scalp, respectively. We have to presume that the basic disturbance is in the blood vessel itself, in that it is more reactive than normal to any noxious influence or to any sudden change in its environment.

In some patients the headache may alternate from one side of the head to the other. Why this changing sensitivity? Some scientists have shown that cells around the blood vessels, known as mast cells, release granules at the time of migraine headache. These granules contain histamine and heparin (a substance which diminishes the clotting power of the blood). It is thought that histamine and heparin play a part in producing pain and tenderness in the artery affected by migraine so that a certain time must elapse before another attack can occur on that side to permit the building up of further granules. In that way the site of the attack may vary from side to side. There is a "refractory period" after most attacks of migraine. A person who avoids red wine because it induces migraine headache may find that he or she can drink it for several days or weeks immediately after he or she has suffered an attack. The vessels appear to have exhausted their capability of reacting for a certain period.

We have then the picture of overreactive vessels. A sudden blow to the head may stimulate the sequence of constriction and dilatation by direct action on the vessels. An emotional shock may induce an attack within minutes, possibly by chemical agents circulating in the blood stream. Chemicals in food or wine may act directly on blood vessels or again set off some intermediate reaction that sets the migraine process in motion. The sudden drop in the female hormone estrogen at the time of menstruation may induce the changes through blood chemicals. The chemicals in question are very likely to be serotonin and prostaglandin E_1 in the circulating blood, and bradykinin and histamine in the vicinity of the dilated scalp arteries.

When faced with such a complex disease, is it any wonder that we have so many treatments for migraine but no cure? Treatments range through psychotherapy, acupuncture, manipulation of the neck, diets of apple cider, vinegar, and wild honey, and a variety of medicines. We cannot replace the patients' vessels with ones that will not react so briskly, but we may be able to desensitize them. We cannot cure migraine, but we can provide relief for the majority of patients with this distressing ailment. A discussion of the various approaches to therapy follows in the next chapter.

11
The Treatment of Migraine

In treating migraine we are struggling with an octopus in murky waters. It is easy to identify the tentacles and even to lop off one or two of them, but where is the heart of the beast?

It is likely that future research will show some specific defect in the blood vessels of migraine patients which leaves them vulnerable to the influence of many internal and external stimuli. Our present treatment is to reduce the number of such stimuli and to attempt to reduce the changes in the cranial blood vessels by specific medication. There are many who never seek attention for their headaches because they believe that nothing can be done to help them. There are others who believe that if they take a pill whenever a headache becomes too severe, they have done all that is humanly possible, whether it works or not, and that they must then put up with their headache for hours or even days at a time. Much is known about migraine and much can be done about it. Migraine does not destroy life but it can destroy the joy of living. Treatment starts with the consideration of the patient as well as the disease.

A PATIENT IS A PERSON

We have seen that the migraine patient is not subject to more stresses than other people but reacts more strongly to them. While there may be some advantage in reducing the stresses from without, the logical approach is to try to strengthen the resistance to stress from within. It is first necessary for the patient to know himself or herself, to stand back and view himself or herself objectively.

What are your internal resources, your strong points, and are you using them to the best advantage? Are you using your abilities to help others in the family and in the community or are you swamping them in self-pity because you are concentrating only on your inadequacies, your illness, and your disappointments? Do you have a clear goal in life, one worth achieving? If so, do you have ability to achieve it? Is it a realistic goal? Will it give you happiness and bring happiness to others? What is the most logical approach to success, and how can you best work toward it? Some time spent occasionally in this form of constructive introspection may save much time and trouble in the long run. There is the well-known story of the airplane captain who announced that he had bad news. "The navigator has lost his way and we do not know where we are going. However I also have good news. We have a tail-wind and are making excellent progress."

We must live in the present, work in the present, and, to the best of our ability, enjoy doing so. But the present must also be used for planning an acceptable future. I believe that everyone must have some sort of goal. To live for the day is not enough for most people. If there is no joy in the daily routine, why isn't there? In what way can it be changed? Would a different job, a different environment for living or working, a different approach to life give you the stimulus you are seeking?

There must always be something to look forward to, apart from the mere hope of survival. There are times, of course, when difficulties appear in such profusion that it is possible only to tackle each day as it comes.

Then, when things ease up a little, the time comes again for further stock-taking, a renewal of motivation, and an upsurge of activity. Along with the broad view of the future, there must be some resting places along the way, some small pleasures to enliven each day or each week. If you are one of those people who never take time off for a hobby, an afternoon away from the children, or a quiet drink at the end of the day, if you never exercise, go to the movies, or plan a vacation, you are deliberately closing off the safety valve which would prevent the internal pressure from rising to dangerous levels. This applies to women as well as men, particularly women with small children who may feel permanently house-bound, without any little breaks from routine and with few of the daily contacts which provide variety for those men and women working in the world outside the home.

Finally, the process of introspection must include one's personal inadequacies. In what way do you not measure up to your own expectations and those of your husband or wife, children, and friends? If there is some serious personal problem involving social, sexual, or business relationships, or just coping with general daily chores, you would benefit from discussing these with your family doctor. He may refer you to a psychiatrist. There is no need to feel apprehensive about visiting a psychiatrist if this is recommended. Only a small proportion of a psychiatrist's work deals with those who have serious mental illness. Most of their patients are seeking the guidance for emotional problems or for symptoms of anxiety and depression which a psychiatrist is skilled in providing. Discussing a problem, particularly with someone trained in counseling, may reveal a solution which has not occurred to you. If there are a series of minor problems which are a recurring cause of anxiety, analyzing them will help you learn to cope with them one at a time. If the problem is beyond your own resources, you may be helped by formal psychotherapy.

The results of an interesting combined approach have been reported by Sydney psychologists K. R. and D. M. Mitchell in the treatment of patients with migraine. They started with the premise that the reduction of migraine frequency depended upon the ability to control emotional reactions, and they prepared two programs to compare their effectiveness. In the first program, relaxation training was followed by the application of this training to the tension-producing situations peculiar to the individual. The second treatment group went on to desensitization procedures which included making a graded list of anxiety-producing stimuli, evoking these by imagery, and pairing each stimulus with a relaxed state. A further stage was "assertive therapy," in which the subjects underwent training in acting out their feelings of love, affection, or hostility in socially acceptable and appropriate forms. Various difficulties, such as sexual problems, were explained and discussed. While the level of anxiety did not drop appreciably during the thirty-two-week treatment period, the last group with combined relaxation, desensitization, and assertive therapy showed significant reduction in the frequency and severity of migraine attacks in contrast to the other group.

Patients may be helped by any means of relaxation of mind and body. Some may benefit from yoga or transcendental meditation. There is little doubt that the ideal treatment for migraine includes both psychological and physical measures.

THE WAY OF LIFE

The common factor in the wide variety of precipitants of migraine appears to be the *rate of change* within the body or its environment. This can be as direct as a blow on the head or as indirect as sleeping late on Sunday morning. If the only aim in life were to prevent migraine, either a life of unrelieved monotony or one maintained at a steady pitch of feverish excitement would be the solution. Since neither is practical nor desirable, some compromise has to be worked out, avoiding as far as possible sudden peaks and troughs in emotional tone. This is largely a matter of common sense *and planning.* The working day should be organized to run as smoothly as possible, with the work load spread evenly over each day and over each week. On the weekend, there is no need to let everything slump. A radical change of pace from constant tension to complete relaxation is a sure way to ensure that the weekend is spoiled by a headache. Sleeping in is a particularly pernicious habit for many and is to be avoided by all prone to "weekend migraine."

Anything found to be a trigger factor should obviously be eliminated whenever possible. Missing meals, drinking red wines, or eating certain foods affect only certain people, and each individual must find out which, if any, of these factors applies to him or her. There are many people who scrupulously abstain from eating chocolates, fatty foods, and oranges simply because they have heard that they are "bad for migraine." They are not necessarily bad for migraine except for that person who has a sensitivity to them, physical or psychological, inherent or conditioned. A few people get their headaches only after severe exercise, but this does not mean that all exercise is forbidden. On the contrary, regular exercise accustoms the blood vessels to a normal sequence of dilatation rather than the incongruous combination of dilatation and constriction which is responsible for migraine. It has been said that standing on the head induces a reflex vasoconstriction of scalp arteries which is beneficial in migraine and which may actually abort an attack if the patient is astute enough to detect the early symptoms, agile enough to stand on his or her head, and devoid of the embarrassment which this custom may cause!

PHYSICAL MEASURES

What physical treatment may be helpful? The age-old method of massaging the scalp or neck muscles, which contract reflexly in migraine, often gives considerable relief. Relaxation exercises (outlined in Chapter 7) will also help in reducing the frequency of migraine attacks. The arteries which supply the scalp run through near the large temporal muscles which control the jaws. In anyone with the habit of jaw-clenching, the constant change in configuration of the jaw muscles distorts the arteries, which may constrict and then undergo rebound dilatation, making them susceptible to the changes of migraine. Any method which aids in relaxation, whether it be formal exercise, yoga, or hypnosis, may decrease the frequency of migraine.

The application of hot or cold packs is another time-honored remedy which merits closer study. In theory, cold packs placed over the large arteries, such as those in the temples, should constrict them and reduce the intensity of the headache. Hot packs are used to dilate the small peripheral vessels to flush the skin and permit the free flow of blood through it (Figure 6). Someone should design an apparatus like a skull cap with a cool band encircling the brow and a warm dome encompassing the head, to see if it compensated for its macabre appearance by its effectiveness in relieving migraine headache.

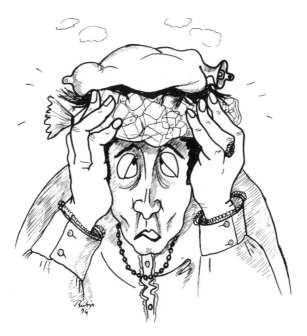

Figure 6. A home treatment for migraine headache. Some people say that their headache is eased by applying heat and others swear by ice packs. Both can be right. Ice cubes applied to the large arteries in the temples, forehead, and neck will make them constrict, thus reducing blood flow and pain. Heating the small blood vessels of the scalp will cause them to dilate, allowing blood to flow more freely out of the tender large arteries. The lady in the illustration is shrewder than she looks.

MANIPULATION, ACUPUNCTURE, AND SURGERY

The question of the treatment of migraine never comes up for discussion without someone claiming that manipulation of the neck is an infallible cure. Certainly any cervical disturbances should be adequately treated, just as it is important to eliminate any other known trigger factor in migraine. My own experience is that manipulation of the neck benefits only a limited number of patients. Many of the patients whom I see have already had their necks manipulated by doctors or chiropractors without any significant change in their headache pattern. Doctor James Cyriax of London, one of the most objective of the observers in this field, has stated that "an attack of migraine can sometimes be instantly aborted by strong traction on the neck. Half a minute's traction in some cases is regularly successful, in others not." He goes on to say, "A minority of patients have reported to me, some years after the reduction by manipulation of a cervical disk, that since that time attacks of obvious migraine have ceased." He noted such improvement only in middle-aged patients—not in the young. I remain skeptical about any specific role for neck disturbance in migraine and the advantages to be obtained from manipulating it.

Neck manipulation is currently being supplanted in popular appeal by the traditional Chinese method of acupuncture. The nerve impulses set up by acupuncture needles can partly suppress the perception of pain. It is conceivable that this could help to relieve the pain of migraine. It is difficult at this time to see how it could prevent or cure migraine in the long term. Nor has it done so in any migraine patient of my acquaintance, although I have had some patients with tension headache improve substantially during a course of acupuncture, only to relapse later.

The same lack of success must be reported for all surgical procedures devised over the last five decades. Operations to divide various nerves and arteries in the head and neck may give a temporary respite from migraine but no permanent benefit. There is a case for tying off and sectioning a scalp artery if it is habitually, and apparently selectively, involved by migraine, particularly one which has been damaged by head injury. It is a simple procedure and may at least give some period of freedom from headache.

HISTAMINE SENSITIZATION

An old method of treating migraine is to give increasing doses of histamine, a potent dilator of cranial arteries, in the hope of desensitizing them to other dilator influences. Unfortunately, histamine acts on the intracranial arteries more than on the scalp arteries, which are the ones largely responsible for the migraine headache. There is no evidence that a general release of histamine causes migraine, but the histamine level does increase slightly in the blood after the attack, suggesting that it may be released locally at the site of headache. The antihistamine drugs in present use do little to prevent migraine. A new group of antihistamines which block histamine-2 receptors (a different histamine action on blood vessels) is now being studied.

The technique of histamine desensitization involves daily injections of histamine, increasing progressively in strength, or three intravenous infusions at weekly intervals. (An infusion is a slow injection of a solution into a vein by a drip apparatus given over a period of hours.) The latter method has the advantage that the patient's reaction can be observed closely. The object is to run the intravenous drip at a speed sufficient to induce flushing of the face but not enough to provoke headache. When Dr. George Selby and I analyzed results of this treatment in the 1960s, we found after eight months that 21 percent of the patients had remained free of headache and 42 percent were substantially improved. It is questionable whether the results warrant the time and inconvenience involved, but it can be used for patients not responding to other treatments.

HORMONAL THERAPY AND FLUID RETENTION

Because of the fluid and salt retention that coincides with migraine, and which can also be a prominent feature in the days preceding menstruation, salt restriction has been advocated, along with drugs called diuretics which help eliminate salt from the body. Fluid and salt retention can certainly be prevented, and this may relieve unpleasant symptoms such as distension of the abdomen and swelling of the face, fingers, and ankles. Regrettably, it does not usually prevent migraine.

The discovery that the fall in estrogen levels initiates premenstrual migraine has renewed interest in the possibilities of hormonal treatment. Different doses, combinations, and sequences of synthetic estrogens and progesterones have been used in the various forms of the contraceptive pill, and these have been tried to see if premenstrual migraine might be abolished. While it is true that some pills give rise to less headache than others and that the occasional patient may lose her headaches on a particular pill, the majority find that menstrual migraine continues to appear predictably. Treatment with synthetic progestogenic agents have proved disappointing.

A long-standing treatment which does seem to help some patients is the twice-weekly injection of a hormone which stimulates the ovaries, called chorionic gonadotrophin. We have given chorionic gonadotrophic hormone, but only about 40 percent of the patients showed worthwhile improvement. This same proportion of patients improves with any new form of treatment, particularly when supported by regular visits to a doctor. Further work is required before any form of hormone therapy can be recommended with confidence.

STOPPING THE ACUTE ATTACK

If migraine recurs only infrequently or if it appears at predictable times, such as the day before menstruation starts or Sunday morning when lying in bed, then it is simple enough to take the appropriate medication at the first symptom of an attack. When a sufferer awakens regularly with a fully developed headache, its occurrence can often be analyzed and prevented in the future by taking a pill the night before. This can be done if the patient predictably feels elated the day before an attack or has some other identifiable warning. For children, one or two aspirin usually stops the attack from progressing, but there are few adults whose attacks will be halted by any of the commonly used analgesics, including some combinations that have been marketed under brand names which suggest that they are specifically for migraine.

Most of the pills prescribed by doctors for treatment of the acute attack of migraine are not pain killers but contain ergotamine tartrate, an agent which constricts the large arteries of the scalp and thereby prevents the migraine attack from developing. For this reason, the dose must be suitable for that individual and the pills taken before the arteries are too dilated. Patients must therefore carry the pills with them so that they can take one or two as soon as there is the first symptom of an attack. If each episode starts with blurring of vision or a similar disturbance, the pills should be taken immediately so that their contents have time to constrict the scalp arteries before the situation is irretrievable. If the patient feels nauseated and vomits in the early stages of the attack, there is no point in taking medication orally. Under these circumstances the use of a suppository is logical and effective. Another method which can be used is to inhale a fine powder of ergotamine tartrate deeply into the lungs from a spray or "medihaler."

Some pills consist of ergotamine tartrate alone. Others have caffeine in them because it increases constriction of the arteries as well as acting as a stimulant. A third group contains an additional agent to diminish nausea.

The following are some of those most commonly employed.

Ergotamine tartrate alone

Coated tablets, each containing one milligram (Femergin, Gynergen) or uncoated tablets of one milligram (Lingraine, Ergomar). Every patient has to determine the suitable dose, sufficient to stop the migraine developing but not enough to cause nausea as a side effect. The usual range is from one to three tablets at the first indication of an attack, repeated in one-half to one hour if necessary. If the headache has not been relieved after the repeated dose, there is no virtue in taking more; indeed it can be dangerous because excessive amounts can cause whiteness and numbness of the fingers from constriction of the small vessels. The uncoated tablets are said to be absorbed well from the mouth if held under the tongue but there is some doubt about this and most of the medication is probably absorbed from the stomach. A traditional way of prescribing ergotamine tablets is to direct that the tablet be taken every hour for up to six hours, but this is not really an effective method because the object of the treatment is to induce a rapid constriction of the scalp arteries, best achieved by a large dose given early. The most direct way of accomplishing this is by injection, and some patients who do not respond to tablets or suppositories can be taught to give themselves an injection. By this route the dosage is lower than if given by mouth, one-quarter to one-half milligram by subcutaneous or intramuscular injection.

Compounds containing ergotamine tartrate
Cafergot.   The combination of ergotamine tartrate one milligram with caffeine one hundred milligrams in Cafergot tablets (or Cafergot-Q tablets which may be chewed for more rapid absorption). Two are usually given at the onset of the attack and may be repeated. Some people are sensitive to caffeine and may feel unpleasantly overstimulated if more than two tablets are taken.

Cafergot–PB suppositories.   The suppositories of ergotamine tartrate contain two milligrams of the active agent as well as caffeine. On the first occasion these are used it is advisable to cut one in half (after cooling it in the refrigerator) and insert only one-half since some patients notice cramps in the legs after the full dose contained in the suppository. Once it is established that the suppositories are well tolerated, one may be inserted at the first indication of an attack, and the patient should then lie down for an hour or so until the headache wears off.

Ergodryl. These capsules contain the same ingredients as Cafergot tablets with the addition of diphenhydramine (Benadryl), an antihistamine, and are used in the same way as Cafergot tablets.

Migral or Migril. These contain two milligrams of ergotamine tartrate as well as caffeine and cyclizine as an antiemetic. Because the active agent is double the dose of that in Cafergot and Ergodryl, it is advisable to take only one at the onset of an attack and this may be repeated in one-half to one hour if required.

Some substances other than ergotamine tartrate have been tried in managing the acute episode, but none have gained full acceptance. Some 70 percent of patients find that their attacks subside rapidly with adequate dosage of ergotamine tartrate medication if taken early enough. It is recommended that ergotamine is not taken during pregnancy because it may cause mild contractions of the uterus. I have not known its use in pregnancy to lead to miscarriage or other adverse effect. Indeed, if it were effective as an abortifacient, it would enjoy considerably greater sales than it does as a remedy for migraine. All of these preparations are best kept in reserve for the acute attack and not taken regularly each day. If the frequency of attacks increases, other measures must be taken which are detailed below.

PREVENTING MIGRAINE

It is to be hoped that attention to psychological factors, elimination of precipitating causes, and relaxation exercises will have gone some way toward reducing the frequency and severity of migraine, and that the attacks when they come will be abbreviated by the use of ergotamine preparations. However, the fact must be faced that there are some people whose attacks will continue unabated in spite of these measures. And there are an unfortunate few whose attacks increase until they occur almost daily.

There are still many things that can and should be done. It is important to search for a cause for the increasing intensity of migraine. Among possible causes might be the use of the contraceptive pill, an increase in blood pressure, or the abuse of ergotamine preparations. The term abuse here means that the patient is taking these tablets every day in anticipation of a headache, whether or not one is developing. This custom may lead to a rebound headache as the vessels dilate when the effect of ergotamine wears off. Under these circumstances the doctor may recommend a week in the hospital so that the vicious cycle can be broken. Often if a migraine sufferer can enjoy a short spell isolated from the responsibilities of everyday life while being regimented by the protective hospital routine, he or she can be freed of migraine and permanently change the old pattern. The other important possible causes to be considered are the onset of a depressive state, which may require treatment with antidepressant tablets as well as psychological support, and an increase in emotional strain.

There are a number of medications which have proven their value in reducing the frequency of migraine attacks when taken two or three times a day as a preventitive measure. First among these are the "antiserotonin" substances. These agents block the direct effect of serotonin on the blood vessels, where it could be responsible for constriction of the smaller arteries and their branches and for sensitizing the vessels to cause pain. One of these agents, methysergide, also increases the effect of any circulating substance that maintains tone in the larger arteries. Thus, it has a two-fold action in preventing migraine.

Methysergide (Sansert, Deseril) is among the most efficient of all prophylactic agents for migraine. It has the disadvantage that about one-third of all those who take it for the first time experience aching of the arms or legs, indigestion, or other odd symptoms for the first few days. Most of these symptoms disappear fairly rapidly, but there remain some 10 percent of patients who cannot tolerate it. Of the other 90 percent, the majority either lose their headaches entirely or experience less than half the previous frequency. If ergotamine preparations have to be used to treat these attacks which occur in spite of methysergide, they are usually more effective in getting rid of the headache than they were before. It is recommended that dosage starts with one tablet three times daily, and I would suggest that on the first occasion a tablet be broken in half and taken as a test dose to ensure that it is well tolerated. You must be guided by your doctor as to the maximum dose to be taken. Once improvement of the headache is established, the dose can be reduced to the minimum necessary to keep the attacks under control. Sometimes only one or two tablets each night may be sufficient to maintain improvement.

In the early days of methysergide treatment, when large doses were given continuously, some patients developed abdominal or chest pain caused by the excessive growth of fibrous tissue. Although this naturally gave rise to concern, it could be reversed by stopping treatment. Nowadays it is recommended that the pills be stopped altogether for one month in every four to prevent the development of fibrotic side effects. Occasionally treatment may cause little veins of the cheeks and nose to become more prominent but this is uncommon. The appetite may increase and some patients put on weight when taking methysergide, but this applies to many effective migraine remedies. If several vomiting days are replaced by several eating days each week, it is hard to avoid the tendency to gain weight—except by a general reduction of food intake spread over the whole week. Like the ergotamine preparations, methysergide may occasionally cause whiteness and numbness of the fingers or signs of constriction of vessels elsewhere. If so, this should be discussed at once with your doctor. The treatment may have to be stopped or used in combination with other tablets which block this excessive constrictor action, such as hydergine.

Other antiserotonin agents, such as pizotifen (Sandomigran, BC105) or cyproheptadine (Periactin), are also useful in preventing migraine in the dose of one to two tablets three times daily. They may cause some drowsiness in the early stages and may also stimulate the appetite so that weight-watching becomes necessary, but this is a small price to pay for freedom from headache in those in whom it is successful. Falling out of the hair is a side effect which is often quoted as a disadvantage of the antiserotonin agents. With all the preparations we have tried, whether they be antiserotonin agents or not, periodic falling out of the hair has been noted by 1 percent. It seems probable that at any one time 1 percent of the female population is undergoing a molting season. The hair may become a little thin, but in my experience it has always grown again normally whether or not the pills are continued.

Other sorts of pills such as clonidine and agents known as beta-blockers (they block one of the actions of adrenaline) have also been used. They are effective in patients with the combination of migraine and high blood pressure. They can also block some of the effects of anxiety, but their action in migraine alone varies from patient to patient. Some chemical relatives of ergotamine also find a place in the prevention of migraine, particularly those with a mild prolonged tonic constrictor effect on blood vessels such as dihydroergotamine (DHE).

Finally, the group of drugs known as the monoamine oxidase (MAO) inhibitors have also been used with success in migraine. Because they require some restriction of diet, including the elimination of cheese and red wine, they are not altogether popular but can be kept in reserve for the patient who has tried everything and still continues to suffer from migraine. Foods which should not be eaten while taking MAO inhibitors, such as phenelzine, include meat extracts, broad beans, pickled herring, and chicken livers, as well as cheese and red wines. No other medication should be taken at the same time without discussing it with your doctor.

WHAT OF THE FUTURE?

There is no one sure cure for migraine. Work is continuing in laboratories in many parts of the world. Scientists are studying the blood vessels themselves, their reactions to various chemical substances and to stimulation of their nerve supply, as well as the effects of pharmaceutical agents. Others are examining the psychological basis of migraine and various physical factors which can affect the mind and, through it, the body. There is certainly great hope that in the future migraine can be removed from the list of scourges which make life unhappy for so many people. In the meantime much can be done with the tools we already possess, but it requires a conscientious and sustained effort by both patient and doctor.

12
Cluster Headache (Migrainous Neuralgia)

This chapter might well be labeled "for men only" since cluster headache is an exception to the feminine dominance of the headache problem. Some 85 percent of all those affected by cluster headache are males. This headache has a curious intermittent pattern of bouts or clusters of intensely severe pains which recur once, twice, or even up to ten times in twenty-four hours and continue for weeks or months. The pain then disappears in eight out of ten patients and goes into recess for months or years. It then comes back with its previous intensity for another devastating bout. There is no known cause for each attack. The condition is often confused with tic douloureux because of the severity of the pain but unlike tic, which strikes with stabs as brief as a lightning flash, the pains in cluster headache last from ten minutes to several hours at a time. It is also confused with migraine, hence the alternative term "migrainous neuralgia" which is still favored in Britain. In about 20 percent of all patients the pains recur regularly, without intermission, more in the manner of migraine. This is now called "chronic cluster headache."

The condition was first described in 1840 by Moritz H. Romberg, then Professor of Medicine at the University of Berlin, a fact forgotten by English-speaking authors who usually attribute its discovery to Dr. Wilfred Harris of London in 1926. Romberg used the term "ciliary neuralgia" because "ciliary" means related to the eyes or the eyelashes and the pain of cluster headache usually centers around the eye. He wrote: "The pupil is contracted. The pain not unfrequently extends over the head and face. The eye generally weeps and becomes red. The symptoms occur in paroxysms, of a uniform or irregular character, and isolated or combined with facial neuralgia and hemicrania." Romberg considered that it might be caused by tuberculosis of the glands in the neck which was a common disease at that time. He also thought it could be "brought on by discharges, especially seminal emissions" and "the development of puberty" among a long list of irrelevancies. The ones quoted are relevant because cluster headache frequently begins in teenage boys, although the cause of the relationship remains obscure.

The condition was rediscovered and renamed in the 1930s by Dr. B. T. Horton, a physician at the Mayo Clinic, Rochester, Minnesota. Doctor Horton and his colleagues believed cluster headache was caused by the release of histamine, called it histaminic cephalgia, and treated it by histamine desensitization. Doctor Michael Anthony working in our laboratories has now shown that histamine is indeed released during the pain of cluster headache. Horton's hypothesis may yet prove to be correct.

The term in current use, "cluster headache," was coined by Dr. Charles Kunkle (now of Portland, Maine) and his colleagues in 1954.

A UNIQUE HEADACHE PATTERN

Once encountered, the pain of cluster headache is unlikely to be confused with anything else. The pain is invariably one-sided and usually sticks to the same side of the head, although there have been instances of it changing from one side to another in the middle of a bout. It is felt deeply behind one eye in 60 percent of the patients but commonly radiates to the forehead, temple, cheek, and upper gum on the same side of the face. The nostril on that side may ache and burn and usually is blocked or runs with fluid. Sometimes the palate may also be involved and aching may spread to the lower gum, jaw, ear, or even the neck.

The pain of cluster headache is usually extraordinarily severe once the bout is established. The patient may leap to his feet and stride up and down holding his hand over his eye. More temperate descriptions of the pain include adjectives like "burning, boring, piercing, tearing, and screwing." The pain usually comes on suddenly, lasts for ten minutes to two hours, and then dies away. It usually returns two or three times in the twenty-four hours, commonly awakening the patient from sleep. This distressing complaint continues with its diabolical periodicity, often recurring at the same time in every day and night for a period of two to eight weeks and occasionally longer. It then mercifully remits, only to recur months or years later. The average frequency in our patients was one bout per year, but many had two each year and an unfortunate few suffered three or four bouts in every year. At the other end of the scale, some patients had intervals of freedom of three to four years between bouts.

The disorder usually develops between the ages of ten and thirty, although we have known patients to experience it for the first time even in old age.

SOME CURIOUS ASPECTS

As the pain becomes severe, the eye on the affected side becomes bloodshot and often waters. The eyelid droops and the pupil often constricts, indicating that the sympathetic nerves to the eye are no longer functioning on that side. Vision may become blurred in the affected eye. The nostril blocks or runs on one or both sides. The forehead may flush and sweat, and the patient sometimes feels a little nauseated. The arteries may dilate on the side of the headache as they do in migraine, and the scalp often feels tender to the touch. The eye may appear puffy, and little lumps may be felt inside the mouth like hives.

During the period of a cluster headache, any substance which dilates blood vessels will promptly trigger off an attack. Alcohol is the most universal of these, and the patient may have to abstain totally for the duration. A patient who used carbon tetrachloride in his dry-cleaning business said that inhalation of the fumes would immediately set off an episode of pain. Nitroglycerin has the same effect and so has histamine.

Doctor Karl Ekbom of Stockholm reported a patient with angina pectoris (chest pain from narrowing of the coronary arteries) whose chest pain almost disappeared during several bouts of cluster headache, although he maintained the same exercise load. Some vasodilator substance, such as histamine, circulating in the blood stream during cluster headache could account for this observation. There is also an increased incidence of peptic ulcer in cluster patients (14 percent of Ekbom's 105 patients and 20 percent of the patients of Dr. John Graham of Boston), which may well be related to the release of histamine since it stimulates gastric secretion.

There is only rarely a family history of cluster headache. Doctor Graham has drawn attention to the distinctive facial appearance of many patients subject to cluster headache—a furrowed thick skin with a ruddy complexion.

IS THIS A VARIATION OF MIGRAINE?

There are certainly many similarities between the symptoms of migraine and of cluster headache, but the differences are even more striking. Cluster headache is much less common than migraine in a proportion of about one to twenty. Cluster headache affects males predominantly, while migraine is more common in women. Cluster headache rarely starts in childhood—one of our patients had one single brief pain at the age of eight—while it is quite usual for migraine to start under the age of ten. It is possible for patients to suffer from both disorders. One patient of mine had the extraordinary and unpleasant experience of having a bout of cluster headache overlap with an increased frequency of migraine attacks, one affecting the left side of his head and the other the right. He was never in any doubt about the different characteristics of the two types of pain. Cluster headache is almost invariably unilateral while migraine may spread to both sides of the head or be bilateral from the start. The focal neurological symptoms which are so often a part of the migraine attack—the flashing lights in front of the eyes, pins and needles, and other sensations—are extremely rare in cluster headache.

Finally, the biochemical changes which have been found in our laboratory appear to demarcate the two conditions just as clearly as does the clinical pattern. Blood serotonin drops sharply in migraine but does not alter in cluster headache. Blood histamine elevates sharply in cluster headache, but in migraine a small increase becomes apparent only at the conclusion of an attack.

CAUSES OF CLUSTER HEADACHE

Some recent studies have clarified our views as to what is going on in cluster headache although we still don't understand the cause. Doctor B. J. Horton first drew attention to the fact that the skin temperature increased on the side of the headache, associated with the flushing of the skin that gave origin to an old term "red migraine." We have examined five patients during an attack of cluster headache by thermography, a photographic technique that records the amount of heat given off from each skin area. Two of our patients showed a cold spot over one eye as the pain first began. This later disappeared as the pain intensified, and "hot spots" appeared in the temple, nose, and cheek on the side of the pain. Another patient also became warmer on the affected side, and the other two showed little change. Doctor Arnold P. Friedman (lately of New York, now in Tucson, Arizona) and his colleagues have examined a large number of patients with cluster headache between attacks and have noted small cold spots standing out like islands on the side of the forehead habitually affected by the headache. These were in the same areas that initially became cold during the attack in our patients. This suggests that there is some abnormality in the small branches of the blood vessels of the forehead in the patients with cluster headache.

There has been only one case recorded of an arteriogram being done at the time of the pain. Doctors Karl Ekbom and T. Greitz of Stockholm demonstrated that the internal carotid artery was narrowed just after it entered the skull, and the appearance suggested that the wall of the artery had become thickened and swollen. Since Dr. Michael Anthony has shown that histamine is released in cluster headache, it is tempting to try to put these facts together. We know that histamine is released in various allergies, such as hives. Could histamine release cause "hives of the carotid artery" so that its wall becomes swollen? This would certainly explain the pain of cluster headache felt deeply behind the eye, because the wall of the carotid artery contains a rich network of nerves which would be compressed by swelling of the artery wall, and it is known that this part of the artery refers pain to the eye. It would also explain the drooping eyelid and small pupil because the nerves responsible for maintaining tone in the muscle of the upper eyelid and for enlarging the pupil of the eye travel in the wall of the carotid artery.

The sequence of events could thus be caused by the release of histamine into the common carotid artery from an unknown source. Histamine could also cause flushing of the face, pain, and sensitivity to touch.

Cluster headache does not seem to be a conventional allergic reaction. There was no consistent seasonal link in our patients even though some were susceptible to their bouts at the same time of each year. The seasonal incidence was equally distributed among spring, summer, fall, and winter.

TREATING EACH CLUSTER AS IT COMES

As with migraine, various surgical approaches to the problem have been tried. Blockade or section of the head and neck nerves has been undertaken unsuccessfully. Cutting the trigeminal nerve which supplies the face with sensation will prevent the pain of the disorder, but at the expense of the face remaining numb permanently.

Antihistamine tablets have been used without much success. These substances will block some actions of histamine when it is freely circulating but not when it is absorbed into tissues, such as the internal carotid artery. A new series of agents which block other actions of histamine are now under investigation.

The present approach to treatment is much the same as for migraine, but with the important difference that the pills or injections must be given in advance of the anticipated pain so that the vessels are constricted before they can react to any dilator substance such as histamine. Tablets of methysergide can be given regularly during a bout of cluster headache.

Ergotamine tartrate pills may also be taken morning and night for the duration of the bout. If this is not effective, it may be given by injection, the time of injection varying so that it precedes the usual onset of the attacks of pain.

With one or another of these regimes, most patients can be kept free of pain until the bout subsides spontaneously. The pills or injections can be stopped for a day when it is calculated that the bout should have ended. If another attack then occurs, the same routine can be adopted for a further week, until the bout has ceased. Then it is to be hoped that there will be a long remission until the same treatment is required for the next round.

Psychological factors are less apparent in the early stages of cluster headache than they are in migraine, but eventually many patients may understandably become depressed and require treatment for depression.

In 1840 Romberg gave some interesting advice. "The eye should be protected by shades, broad brims to the hats or caps, or by blue spectacles. Variety in the mode of exercising the organs is desirable: people who are accustomed to work, requiring a close proximity of the objects to the eye, should exchange it for an occupation allowing a long range of vision; looking upon green fields, residence in pure dry air. The use of the cold bath, and sponging, are also beneficial."

13
You and Your Doctor

The most important ally a headache patient can have is a sympathetic general practitioner who knows the patient, his or her family, and his or her problems as a basis for coming to grips with the headache itself. This presupposes that the family doctor has sufficient time to spend with patients who require it and is familiar with the advances which have been made in the classification, diagnosis, and treatment of headaches over recent years. It may seem that this is looking for perfection, and yet this sort of understanding and guidance is still to be found in this hurried age. Long may it be preserved! The emphasis is placed on the general practitioner because no end of trouble can arise from patients taking themselves to one specialist after another without being referred by their family doctor. Someone has to hold the reins. Someone has to correlate reports from specialists and apply their findings to the best advantage. It is conceivable that a patient with headache could consult an eye doctor who prescribed glasses, then an ear, nose, and throat doctor who fixed up his or her sinus trouble, followed by an orthopedic surgeon who treated a cervical disk disturbance, and so on, while the headache continued unabated. Fortunately, this is not very likely because most specialists realize immediately whether or not a problem lies within their province. However, the family general practitioner is in the best possible position to assess whether one of these specialists or a general physician, neurologist, or psychiatrist would be of the most assistance to each individual case. It may well be that your G. P. takes a particular interest in headache problems himself and can set you on the right road without the need to see a consultant. The important principle is that there must be one doctor who is *your* doctor, who has your interests at heart, and who will do his best to get to the bottom of the trouble and help you to overcome it.

PLEASE HAVE YOUR SYMPTOMS READY

There is a story that a frazzled general practitioner placed a sign in his waiting room saying, "Please have your symptoms ready." It is quite surprising, even in consultant practice when patients may have booked their appointments weeks or more ahead for the sole purpose of discussing their headache problem, to find that some have made no attempt to organize their own thoughts on the subject and may not be able to answer simple direct questions about it. If the doctor asks how long you have had your headache, he is after an approximation and is not usually concerned about the precise day, week, or month. It is rather disconcerting for him to receive the reply, "I really have no idea," when in fact the patient is the only person who can possibly know. For this reason I would recommend making brief notes of the salient features so that the pattern of headache becomes clear to you and your doctor. It is no help to cover sheet after sheet of foolscap with closely spaced writing in order to hand it triumphantly to your doctor as you sit down. The man or woman with interminable memoirs, written or spoken, can impede the progress of the consultation even more effectively than the laconic replies of the uncommunicative patient. The simplest thing is to present to the doctor the symptoms which concern you, their duration, their pattern of recurrence, and the things that you have found make them worse or better. After this, the doctor will probably want certain other specific information. Every doctor has a slightly different approach. Some prefer to ask leading questions throughout. Others like the patient to tell the story in his or her own words. Most combine the two methods. Whatever the approach, there is an obvious advantage if you have your thoughts marshaled before the consultation begins.

THE PATTERN OF HEADACHE

Throughout this book the emphasis has been on diagnosis from the clinical history. Only rarely are special tests required to confirm or deny a certain hypothesis. If the story is presented clearly, the diagnosis will usually become evident as it progresses. Some basic information is required, and the following headings will help you to "have your symptoms ready."

How long have you suffered from headache? Days, weeks, months, or years?

How often does the headache recur? Once a year, once a month, several times a week, or daily?

How long does the headache last? Minutes, hours, or days? Please correlate this with the preceding question. Patients sometimes say that they have, say, three headaches a week, each lasting three days, when what they mean is that the one weekly headache lasts for three days and they then have a break for three or four days before the next one starts.

Is there any pattern about the recurrence of the headache? Does it go away for months at a time, then return in the manner of cluster headache? Has it increased in frequency or changed its pattern lately? Are there two or more varieties of headache which should be analyzed separately? For example, migraine and tension headache may coexist so that the daily dull ache caused by muscle contraction may be punctuated by more severe episodes of migraine.

What area of the head is affected? Both sides or one side only? Right or left or alternating? Is it just one part of the head (forehead, temple, or the back of the head), or is it all over the head? Does it radiate down the neck or elsewhere?

What is the quality of the pain? Is it constant or fluctuating, dull or severe? Does it throb (intensify with each beat of the pulse)?

What is the beginning like? Is the headache present on waking in the morning, or does it waken you from sleep in the middle of the night? Does it come on during the day? If so, are there any warning symptoms, such as visual or other sensory disturbances or a change of mood?

What are the associated features? Do you feel nauseated, vomit, or pass loose bowel movements? Does light hurt your eyes, or does noise worry you? This list of questions could be extended almost indefinitely by referring to the sections dealing with each variety of headache.

Are there any precipitating factors? Does the headache come on at moments of emotional disturbance or nervous tension or at times of relaxation, such as weekends? Does it recur at any particular phase of the menstrual cycle? Is it related to physical exercise, to the taking of certain foods or alcohol, or any other known cause?

Are there any aggravating factors? Is the headache made worse by sudden movement of the head or neck? Is it worse on coughing, sneezing, or straining? Is it worse when standing or when lying down?

Are there any relieving factors? Do hot or cold packs or any other physical measures help? Will the headache go away if you lie down and sleep? Is it eased by ordinary analgesics such as aspirin, phenacetin, or paracetamol, or by stronger tablets containing codeine? Does it ever require injections given by your doctor?

Have you had any other treatment for an acute attack of headache? What were they, and did they stop the headache?

Have you had regular medication of any sort in an attempt to prevent the headache completely? If so, what was the result?

Have you had any other treatment—manipulation of the neck, physiotherapy, acupuncture, or psychotherapy?

HELPING YOUR DOCTOR

Once your doctor has a clear and concise picture of your type of headache, he or she will probably ask about your general health, your past health (with particular reference to head injuries), your family history (with emphasis on headache of any sort), and your personal background. Be honest in your description of smoking habits, alcohol, and your use of any other drugs. Discuss frankly any fear or anxiety which is troubling you, and do not hesitate to bring up sexual problems if there are any. What may seem to be a very grave, embarrassing, or insuperable problem to you could well be one which your doctor has encountered many times before and which may be overcome with the right advice. If you have some particular worry you wish to discuss, bring it up early in the interview so there is time to go into it.

Be honest with yourself and with your doctor about

any symptoms of depression, because these may be responsible for daily headaches or can develop as a reaction to frequent headache. In either event, the vicious circle can often be broken by the relief of depression, and there are now many ways of doing this pharmacologically as well as psychologically.

You can help your doctor by presenting your symptoms logically and briefly and by replying as clearly as possible to his or her questions. Since the doctor's diagnosis depends upon his or her analysis of the history that you give, the whole thing is a collaborative venture. Ideally you know your doctor and have confidence in him or her. He or she respects you as an individual and is anxious to help you. This is a solid basis on which to build.

HELPING YOURSELF

After reading this book you should have a sound idea of the principles of headache, its diagnosis, and its treatment. It is intended to be a help in interpreting your doctor's advice and in carrying it out.

If your headaches continue after trying a particular form of treatment, do not consult a different doctor immediately. Stay with the one doctor so that he or she can proceed with various treatments in regular sequence. If you go off to another doctor, he or she will probably have to start at the same point as the first and may even prescribe the same treatment unless the doctor knows that you did not respond well to it.

If your own doctor is in doubt about the diagnosis or treatment, he or she can refer you to the most appropriate specialist. No matter how much experience one has, one is often glad of another point of view, a fresh assessment of the case. I find that I greatly appreciate the opinion of my colleagues on many different neurological problems. There are occasions when a newly graduated doctor or a medical student may suddenly hit on something which has escaped those with greater experience and may place the diagnostic key within one's grasp. If this be the case, how much more often must a doctor in the most difficult of all specialties, general practice, be glad of another's opinion.

One final point. If a regime of treatment is prescribed, please give it a fair trial. There is nothing more frustrating to a doctor or patient than agreeing on a course of action which is never carried out or to the doctor prescribing a medication which is never taken. The success of any treatment depends on your own understanding and cooperation as well as your doctor's knowledge and ability.

FREEDOM FROM HEADACHE

There are some forms of headache which can be cured completely. Most can be helped considerably. For the common condition of tension headache, there is so much that can be done by the individual. The treatment depends upon the patient as much as the doctor. The way of life and the mental approach to its problems are as important as medication. There are few forms of headache which will respond to one treatment and one treatment only. Most have many facets, each of which must attract our attention. With migraine as with cluster headache, all the clues seem to be at hand to solve the mystery. I feel optimistic that the next ten years will see further steps forward in the solution of these problems. Even if the complete answer is not obtained, advances in knowledge as great as those of the last ten years will enable treatment to become still more effective, until at last the doctor can offer every patient his or her natural right—freedom from headache.

Thomas Willis in the seventeenth century said, "It has become a proverb as a sign of a most rare and admirable thing, 'that his head did never ake.' "

Glossary

Adrenal glands. Glands situated above the kidneys. The central part (medulla) secretes epinephrine (adrenaline) and norepinephrine (noradrenaline). Both amines circulate in the blood stream and constrict the cranial arteries, as well as increasing blood pressure and pulse rate. The outer part of the gland (cortex) produces cortisone.

Air encephalography. An X-ray technique involving the insertion of about thirty milliliters of air into the cerebrospinal fluid to outline the ventricles and other fluid-containing canals in and around the brain.

Alpha rhythm. The dominant brain rhythm recorded in a normal electroencephalogram, usually eight to ten per second.

Amitriptyline. An antidepressant agent which is useful in the management of tension headache and other types of chronic pain (trade names—Tryptanol, Tryptizol, Laroxyl, Elavil, etc.).

Amyl nitrite. A vasodilator substance occasionally used in the management of angina pectoris and in reducing the spasm of vessels in some cases of migraine.

Analgesics. Substances which relieve pain, such as aspirin, phenacetin, and paracetamol.

Aneurysm. A localized dilatation of an artery in which the wall is weaker than a normal artery and may leak to cause subarachnoid hemorrhage.

Angiogram, arteriogram. A specialized X-ray technique in which a radio-opaque dye is injected into an artery to demonstrate whether or not the blood vessels are normal.

Angioma, arterio-venous malformation. An abnormal collection of blood vessels, analogous to a red birthmark, in which blood passes rapidly from arteries to veins.

Aqueduct A channel in the brain which conveys cerebro-spinal fluid from the third to the fourth ventricle.

Arachnoid. A delicate membrane which surrounds the brain and spinal cord and contains the cerebrospinal fluid.

Atheroma. A fatty deposit in the arterial wall which is a common cause of stroke and coronary occlusion.

Basilar artery. An artery formed by the junction of the two vertebral arteries which supplies the brain-stem. It then divides to form two posterior cerebral arteries which supply the visual cortex.

Basilar migraine. A form of migraine in which the branches of the basilar artery are affected, causing symptoms such as giddiness, loss of balance, faintness, and visual disturbances.

Bradykinin. A peptide released in inflammatory processes, causing dilatation of blood vessels.

Brain-stem. A part of the hindbrain resembling a stem or stalk between the midbrain and spinal cord. It contains the nuclei of most of the cranial nerves as well as vital centers concerned with breathing and maintaining blood pressure.

Carbamazepine. An anticonvulsant drug which reduces the jabbing pains of tic douloureux (trade name—Tegretol).

Carcinoid. A tumor of the gastrointestinal tract which secretes serotonin.

Carotid arteries. Large arteries which course through the neck to supply the greater part of the brain through their anterior and middle cerebral branches.

Cerebrospinal fluid. A clear liquid manufactured by the choroid plexuses in the ventricles of the brain, which circulates around the brain and helps to support and protect it.

Cervical migraine. A type of headache with characteristics similar to basilar migraine said to be caused by spurs of bone compressing the vertebral arteries in their course through the cervical spine.

Cervical spine. The bones (vertebrae) of the neck which enclose the spinal cord. The vertebral arteries lie in a canal within the side projections of the bones.

Choroid plexuses. Capillary networks in the ventricles of the brain which form the cerebrospinal fluid.

Ciliary neuralgia. An old name for cluster headache.

Cluster headache. A type of headache recurring in bouts or clusters. Also called migrainous neuralgia or Horton's histaminic cephalgia.

Computerized transverse axial tomography. A new method of X-ray localization of intracranial structures. A thin beam of X rays scans the head in a series of planes. Minute differences in the absorption of the rays are calculated by computer and displayed as numbers or as a pictorial representation of the intracranial contents in each plane.

Cortisone. A steroid hormone made by the cortex of the adrenal glands. Synthetic forms of this hormone are used in treatment.

Costen's syndrome. Pain radiating over the face from the hinge joint of the jaw in front of the ear, commonly caused by imbalance of the bite and jaw-clenching.

Cranial nerves. Twelve pairs arising from or entering the brain, each pair being concerned with special functions such as the sense of smell (1), vision (2), eye movements (3,4,6), facial sensations and jaw movements (5), facial movement (7), hearing (8), swallowing and speech (9,10), head-turning (11), and tongue movement (12).

Cyproheptadine (Periactin). An agent used in the prevention of migrane.

Diazepam. A tranquilizing, anticonvulsant, and muscle-relaxing agent (trade name—Valium).

Diuretic. An agent which reduces the amount of body fluid by promoting the excretion of salt and water in the urine.

Dura. A firm membrane lining the inner side of the skull.

Edema. Swelling of a tissue caused by excessive fluid in the cells or surrounding tissues.

Electroencephalogram (EEG).   A recording of the electrical activity arising from the brain.

Encephalitis.   A viral infection of the brain.

Epinephrine (adrenaline).   See Adrenal glands.

Ergotamine tartrate.   A chemical agent derived from ergot which constricts the arteries of the scalp and is used for this purpose in the treatment of migraine.

Estrogen.   A female hormone, the blood level of which falls just before menstruation, a trigger factor for premenstrual migraine.

Glaucoma.   Increased pressure within the eyeball.

Glial cells.   Connective tissue cells which lie between the nerve cells of the brain and help to nourish them.

Glioma.   A tumor arising from glial cells.

Glossopharyngeal nerve.   The ninth cranial nerve which supplies sensation to part of the ear and the back of the throat as well as innervating muscles concerned with swallowing.

Glossopharyngeal neuralgia.   Painful jabs of pain in the ear and throat caused by irritation of the glossopharyngeal nerve.

Hemicrania.   An ache involving one-half of the head only.

Hemiplegic migraine.   A form of migraine, commonly hereditary, in which one-half of the body becomes weak.

Heparin.   An anticlotting agent contained in body mast cells.

Herpes zoster.   Shingles. A red rash with blisters developing in the distribution of nerve roots, sometimes followed by pain (postherpetic neuralgia).

Histamine.   An amine contained in mast cells and other tissues which is released in allergic reactions and causes dilatation of cranial blood vessels.

Horton's histaminic cephalgia.   See Cluster headache.

Hydrocephalus.   Increased intracranial pressure caused by obstruction to the flow of cerebrospinal fluid or failure of its absorption.

Indomethacin.   An inhibitor of prostaglandin formation

which is used in the treatment of arthritis and has also been employed in migraine. It can cause a continuous dull headache as a side effect.

Isotope-scanning. The use of radioactive isotopes to detect changes in vascularity of tissues. The most usual form of brain scanning is the injection of isotope into a vein and the recording of the isotope passing up the neck vessels into the brain by a gamma camera (dynamic scanning). Later recordings are taken once the isotope is distributed in the brain tissue (static scanning).

Lumbar puncture. The insertion of a fine needle through the skin of the back (lumbar region) into the fluid-containing sac below the lower end of the spinal cord. The procedure is done under local anesthesia to obtain a sample of the cerebrospinal fluid for analysis, or to inject air or dye for specialized X rays, such as air encephalography.

Mast cells. Cells containing granules of histamine and heparin which surround scalp arteries.

Melanoma. A malignant mole.

Meninges. Membranes of the brain. The dura lines the inner side of the skull, the arachnoid contains the cerebrospinal fluid, and the pia covers the brain surface.

Meningioma. A tumor arising from the meninges.

Meningism. Irritation of the meninges without inflammation.

Meningitis. Inflammation of the meninges, usually caused by bacteria.

Meningoencephalitis. Inflammation of the meninges and brain, usually caused by a virus.

Methysergide. A pharmaceutical agent used in the prevention of migraine (trade names—Sansert, Deseril).

Midbrain. Region of brain between cerebral hemispheres and brain-stem, containing area responsible for maintaining consciousness.

Monoamine oxidase (MAO). An enzyme which breaks down monoamines such as serotonin, epinephrine, and norepinephrine. Another type of MAO breaks down phenylethylamine which is found in chocolate. Drugs which inhibit MAO are used in the treatment of depression as well as migraine.

Myalgia.   Muscle pain.

Neuralgia.   Pain arising from inflammation or compression of nerves.

Norepinephrine.   See Adrenal glands.

Ophthalmoplegic migraine.   Migraine headache associated with double vision caused by weakness of the eye muscles.

Papilledema.   Swelling of the optic nerve head in the eye, which can be seen with an ophthalmoscope and is one sign of raised intracranial pressure.

Phenylethylamine.   An amine present in chocolate which has recently been implicated as a possible trigger for migraine.

Pheochromocytoma.   A tumor of the adrenal gland producing epinephrine and norepinephrine which may be responsible for raising blood pressure.

Photophobia.   Dislike of light.

Pia.   The inner of the three brain membranes (meninges).

Pizotifen.   An agent used in the prevention of migraine (trade name—Sandomigran).

Postherpetic neuralgia.   Pain following herpes zoster (shingles).

Progesterone.   A female hormone which becomes elevated in the blood during the second half of the menstrual cycle and in pregnancy.

Prostaglandins.   A series of complex fatty acids which affect blood vessels among other actions. Originally named because of their association with the prostate gland.

REM sleep.   Rapid eye movement phase of sleep. A periodic lightening of the level of sleep in which eye movement occurs.

Serotonin.   An amine manufactured in the intestinal wall and carried in blood platelets from which it may be released to affect blood vessels. Also found in nerve cells and other tissues.

Steroids. A group of substances which includes cortisone. The term "steroids" is used loosely for natural and synthetic forms of cortisone used in treatment.

Subarachnoid hemorrhage. Bleeding into the cerebrospinal fluid, contained in the space beneath the arachnoid membrane.

Subdural hematoma. Bleeding into the space outside the arachnoid membrane but beneath the dura.

Temporal arteritis. Inflammation of the temporal arteries in the scalp which may also affect other vessels of the scalp, brain, and eye.

Tic douloureux. Severe jabbing pain caused by irritation of the trigeminal nerve.

Tomography. An X-ray beam focussed on a particular layer or plane in order to focus it clearly.

Trauma. Injury.

Trepanning. The operation of making a hole in the skull, particularly applied to primitive medicine.

Trigeminal nerve. The nerve supplying sensation to the face. It has three divisions, hence the name trigeminal ("three born at once").

Trigeminal neuralgia. Pain arising from the trigeminal nerve. Commonly used as a synonym for tic douloureux.

Tyramine. An amine present in some foods which is thought to be a trigger factor in some forms of migraine.

Ultrasound. A beam of high-frequency sound waves used to detect structures within the skull by the "echo" or reflection of the beam from them.

Vasomotor rhinitis. Blockage of the nostrils by swelling of the blood vessels in the mucous membrane of the nose.

Ventricles. Canals within the brain containing the cerebrospinal fluid. There are paired lateral ventricles which open into the third ventricle, from which the fluid passes to the fourth ventricle through the aqueduct.

Ventriculography. Demonstration of the size and position

of the ventricles by an X-ray technique which involves
the injection of air into them.

Vertebral arteries.   Arteries ascending in a canal within the
neck vertebrae which unite to form the basilar artery.

Vertebrobasilar insufficiency. Failure of blood flow
through the vertebral and basilar arteries causing symptoms similar to "basilar migraine."

Vertigo. Giddiness, a sense of movement of the head in
relation to the environment or vice versa.

References

(1) Adams, F., *The Seven Books of Paulus Aegineta* (London: Sydenham Society, 1844)

(2) Adams, F., *The Extant Works of Aretaeus, the Cappadocian* (London: Sydenham Society, 1841)

(3) Adams, F., *The Genuine Works of Hippocrates* (Baltimore: Williams and Wilkins, 1939)

(4) Anderson, B., Jr., Heyman, A., Whalen, R.E., and Saltzmann, H.A., *Migraine-like Phenomena after Decompression from Hyperbaric Environment* (Neurology, Minneapolis, Vol. 15, 1965)

(5) Anthony, Michael, Hinterberger, H., and Lance, James W., *The Possible Relationship of Serotonin to the Migraine Syndrome* in *Research and Clinical Studies in Headache* (New York, Basel: Karger, Vol. 2, 1968)

(6) Anthony, Michael, and Lance, James W., *Monoamine Oxidase Inhibition in the Treatment of Migraine* (Archives of Neurology, Vol. 21, 1969)

(7) Anthony, Michael, and Lance, James W., *Histamine and Serotonin in Cluster Headache* (Archives of Neurology, Vol. 25, 1971)

(8) Balla, John I., and Moraitis, S., *Knights in Armour. A Follow-up Study of Injuries after Legal Settlement* (Medical Journal of Australia, Vol. 2, 1970)

(9) Benson, H., Klemchuk, H.P., and Graham, J.R., *The Usefulness of the Relaxation Response in the Therapy of Headache* (Headache, Vol. 14, 1974)

(10) Bickerstaff, E.R., *Impairment of Consciousness in Migraine* (The Lancet, Vol. 2, 1961)

(11) Bille, Bo., *Migraine in School Children* (Uppsala: Almqvist and Wiksell, 1962)

(12) Blau, J.N., and Cumings, J.N., *Method of Precipitating and Preventing Some Migraine Attacks* (British Medical Journal, Vol. 2, 1966)

(13) Blau, J.N., and Pyke, D.A., *Effect of Diabetes on Migraine* (The Lancet, Vol. 2, 1970)

(14) Brenner, C., Friedman, Arnold P., Merritt, H.H., and Denny-Brown, D.E., *Post-Traumatic Headache* (Journal of Neurosurgery, Vol. 6, 1944)

(15) Brewis, M., Poskanzer, D.C., Rolland, C., and Miller, H., *Neurological Disease in an English City* (Acta Neurologica Scandinavica, Vol. 42, Supplement 24, 1963)

(16) Brindley, G.S., and Lewin, B.S., *The Sensations Produced by Electrical Stimulation of the Visual Cortex* (Journal of Physiology, Vol. 196, 1968)

(17) Carlson, L.A., Ekelund, L-G, and Orö, L., *Clinical and Metabolic Effects of Different Doses of Prostaglandin E in Man* (Acta Medica Scandinavica, Vol. 183, 1968)

(18) Carroll, Lewis, *Alice in Wonderland* (London, Collins, chapter 6)

(19) Carroll, Lewis, *Through the Looking Glass* (London, Collins, chapter 4)

(20) Clarke, G.J.R., and Waters, W.E., *Headache and Migraine in a London General Practice* in *The Epidemiology of Migraine* (Bracknell, Berkshire, England: Boehringer Ingelheim, 1974)

(21) Cleland, John, and Southcott, R.V., *Hypervitaminosis A in the Antarctic in the Australasian Antarctic Expedition of 1911–1914: A Possible Explanation of the Illnesses of Mertz and Mawson* (Medical Journal of Australia, Vol. 1, 1969)

(22) Costen, J.B., *A Syndrome of Ear and Sinus Symptoms Dependent upon Disturbed Function of the Temporomandibular Joint* (Annals of Otology, Rhinology and Laryngology, Vol. 43, 1934)

(23) Critchley, Macdonald, *Migraine from Cappadocia to Queen Square* in *Background to Migraine* (London, Heinemann, Vol. 1, 1967)

(24) Cyriax, James, *Textbook of Orthopaedic Medicine* (London: Cassell, Vol. 1, 1962)

(25) Dalsgaard-Nielsen, J., *Some Aspects of the Epidemiology of Migraine in Denmark* in *Kliniske Aspekter i Migraeneforskningen* (Copenhagen: Nordlundes Bogtrykkeri, 1970)

(26) Dexter, J.D., and Weitzman, E.D., *The Relationship of Nocturnal Headaches to Sleep Stage Patterns* (Neurology, Minneapolis, Vol. 20, 1970).

(27) Drake, Daniel, *A Systematic Treatise, Historical, Epidemiological and Practical on the Principal Diseases of the Interior Valley of North America, as may Appear in the Caucasian, African and Indian and Esquimaux Varieties of its Population* (Cincinnati: W.B. Smith & Co., 1850)

(28) Ekbom, Karl, and Greitz, T., *Carotid Angiography in Cluster Headache* (Acta Radiologica Diagnostica, Vol. 10, 1970)

(29) Ekbom, Karl, *Clinical Aspects of Cluster Headache* (Headache, Vol. 13, 1974)

(30) Ellard, John, *Psychological Reactions to Compensable Injury* (Medical Journal of Australia, Vol. 2, 1970)

(31) Elliott, F.A., *Treatment of Herpes Zoster with High Doses of Prednisone* (Lancet, Vol. 2, 1964)

(32) Engel, G.L., Ferris, E.B., and Romano, J., *Focal Electroencephalographic Changes During the Scotomas of Migraine* (American Journal of Medical Science, Vol. 209, 1945)

(33) Every, R.G., *The Significance of Extreme Mandibular Movements* (Lancet, Vol. 2, 1960)

(34) Friedman, Arnold P., *The Headache in History, Literature and Legend* (Bulletin of the New York Academy of Medicine, Vol. 48, 1972)

(35) Friedman, Arnold P., *The (Infinite) Variety of Migraine: Sandoz Foundation Lecture* in *Background to Migraine. Third Migraine Symposium* (London: Heinemann, 1970)

(36) Friedman, Arnold P., Von Storch, T.J.C., and Merritt, H.H., *Migraine and Tension Headaches. A Clinical Study of Two Thousand Cases* (Neurology, Vol. 4, 1964)

(37) Friedman, Arnold P., Wood, E.H., Rowan, A.J., and Frazier, S.H., Jr., *Observations on Vascular Headache of the Migraine Type* in *Background to Migraine, Fifth Migraine Symposium* (London: Heinemann, 1973)

(38) Gammie, K.M., and Waters, W.E., *Headache and Migraine in a Biscuit Factory* in *The Epidemiology of Migraine* (Bracknell, Berkshire, England; Boehringer Ingelheim, 1974)

(39) Goltman, A.M., *The Mechanism of Migraine* (Journal of Allergy, Vol. 7, 1936)

(40) Graham, John R., *Cluster Headache* (Headache, Vol. 11, 1972)

(41) Granerus, G., Svensson, S-E., and Wetterquist, H., *Histamine in Alcohol Drinks* (The Lancet, Vol. 1, 1969)

(42) Guthrie, D., *A History of Medicine* (New York: Thomas Nelson and Sons Ltd., 1947)

(43) Haas, David C., and Sovner, Robert D., *Migraine Attacks Triggered by Mild Head Trauma, and Their Relation to Certain Post-Traumatic Disorders of Childhood* (Journal of Neurology, Neurosurgery and Psychiatry, Vol. 32, 1969)

(44) Hanington, E., Horn, M., and Wilkinson, M., *Further Observations on the Effects of Tyramine* in *Background to Migraine. Third Migraine Symposium* (London: Heinemann, 1970)

(45) Harris, Wilfred, *Ciliary (Migrainous) Neuralgia and Its Treatment* (British Medical Journal, Vol. 1, 1936)

(46) Henderson, William R., and Raskin, Neil H., *Hot-dog Headache: Individual Susceptibility to Nitrite* (Lancet, Vol. 2, 1972)

(47) Henryk-Gutt, Rita, and Rees, W. Linford, *Psychological Aspects of Migraine* (Journal of Psychosomatic Research, Vol. 17, 1973)

(48) Horton, B.T., MacLean, A.R., and Craig, W. McK., *A New Syndrome of Vascular Headache: Results of Treatment with Histamine: Preliminary Report* (Proceedings of Staff Meetings of Mayo Clinic, Vol. 14, 1939)

(49) Hubel, D.H., and Wiesel, T.N., *Receptive Fields and Functional Architecture of Monkey Striate Cortex* (Journal of Physiology, London, Vol. 195, 1968)

(50) Jacobson, Edmund, *You Must Relax* (New York, Toronto, London. McGraw-Hill, 1962)

(51) Jannetta, Peter J., *Observations of the Etiology of Trigeminal Neuralgia in 100 Consecutive Operative Cases. Definitive Microsurgical Treatment by Relief of Compression-Distortion of the Trigeminal Nerve at the Brain Stem* (Paper delivered at Neurosurgical Congress in Tokyo, Sept. 1973)

(52) Jones, James, *The Ice-Cream Headache and Other Stories* (London; Collins, 1968. Fontana Books, 1971)

(53) Kerr, Frederick W.L., *Evidence for a Peripheral Etiology of Trigeminal Neuralgia* (Journal of Neurosurgery, Vol. 26, 1967)

(54) King, Allen B., and Robinson, Sumner M., *Vascular Headaches of Acute Mountain Sickness* (Aerospace Medicine, August, 1972)

(55) Kunkle, E. Charles, Pfeiffer, J.B., Wilhoit, W.M., and Lamrick, L.W., *Recurrent Brief Headaches in "Cluster" Pattern* (North Carolina Medical Journal, Vol. 15, 1954)

(56) Lance, James W., *Mechanism and Management of Headache* (London, Butterworths, Second Edition, 1973)

(57) Lance, James W., *Headaches Occurring During Sexual Intercourse* (Proceedings of the Australian Association of Neurologists, Vol. 11, 1974)

(58) Lance, James W., and Anthony, Michael, *Some Clinical Aspects of Migraine* (Archives of Neurology, Vol. 15, 1966)

(59) Lance, James W., and Anthony, Michael, *Thermographic Studies in Vascular Headache* (Medical Journal of Australia, Vol. 1, 1971)

(60) Lance James W., and Anthony, Michael, *Migrainous Neuralgia or Cluster Headache?* (Journal of Neurological Sciences, Vol. 13, 1971)

(61) Lance, James W., Curran, D.A., and Anthony, Michael, *Investigations into Mechanism and Management of Chronic Headache* (Medical Journal of Australia, Vol. 2, 1965)

(62) Lashley, K.S., *Patterns of Cerebral Integration Indicated by the Scotomas of Migraine* (Archives of Neurology and Psychiatry, Chicago, Vol. 46, 1941)

(63) Lennox, W.G., and Lennox, M.A., *Epilepsy and Related Disorders* (London: Churchill, Vol. 1, 1960)

(64) Liveing, Edward, *On Megrim, Sick-Headache, and Some Allied Disorders: A Contribution to the Pathology of Nerve-Storms* (London: J. and A. Churchill, 1873)

(65) Major, R.H., *The Papyrus Ebers* (Annals of Medical History, New Series. Vol. 2, 1930)

(66) Martin, M.J., Rome, H.P., and Swenson, W.M., *Muscle-Contraction Headache: A Psychiatric Review* (Research and Clinical Studies in Headache: New York, Basel: Karger. Vol. 1, 1967)

(67) Masters, W.H., and Johnson, V.E., *Human Sexual Response* (Boston, Little Brown & Co., 1966)

(68) Matthews, W.B., *Footballer's Migraine* (British Medical Journal, Vol. 1, 1972)

(69) McHenry, L.C., Jr. (ed.), *Garrison's History of Neurology* (Springfield, Illinois: Charles C. Thomas, 1969)

(70) McNally, Ward, *Smithy: The Kingsford Smith Story* (London: Robert Hale, 1966)

(71) Miller, Henry, *Accident Neurosis* (British Medical Journal, Vol. 1, 1961)

(72) Mitchell, K.R., and Mitchell, D.M., *Migraine: An Exploratory Treatment Application of Programmed Behaviour Therapy Techniques* (Journal of Psychosomatic Research, Vol. 15, 1971)

(73) Moffett, A., Swash, M., and Scott, D.F., *Effect of Tyramine in Migraine: A Double-Blind Study* (Journal of Neurology, Neurosurgery and Psychiatry, Vol. 35, 1972)

(74) Moffett, A.M., Swash, M., and Scott, D.F., *Effect of Chocolate in Migraine: A Double-Blind Study* (Journal of Neurology, Neurosurgery and Psychiatry, Vol. 37, 1974)

(75) Ough, C.S., *Measurement of Histamine in California Wines* (Journal of Agriculture and Food Chemistry, Vol. 19, 1971)

(76) Paulson, G.W., and Klawans, H.L., *Benign Orgasmic Cephalgia* (Headache, Vol. 13, 1974)

(77) Pearce, John, *Insulin Induced Hypoglycaemia in Migraine* (Journal of Neurology, Neurosurgery and Psychiatry, Vol. 34, 1971)

(78) Pickering, G.W., and Hess, W., *Observations on the Mechanism of Headache Produced by Histamine* (Clinical Science, Vol. 1, 1933–4)

(79) Pope, Alexander, *The Rape of the Lock*

(80) Ray, B.S., and Wolff, H.G., *Experimental Studies on Headache. Pain Sensitive Structures of the Head and Their Significance in Headache* (Archives of Surgery, Vol. 41, 1940)

(81) Relander, M., Troupp, H., and Björkesten, G. af., *Controlled Trial of Treatment for Cerebral Concussion* (British Medical Journal, Vol. 2, 1972)

(82) Romberg, Moritz H., *A Manual of Nervous Diseases of Man*, trans. by E.H. Sieveking (London: Sydenham Society, 1840)

(83) Rooke, E.D., *Benign Exertional Headache* (Medical Clinics of North America, Vol. 52, 1968)

(84) Sachs, Oliver W., *Migraine. Evolution of a Common Disorder* (London: Faber and Faber, 1970)

(85) Schaumburg, Herbert H., Byck, R., Gerstl, R., and Mashman, Jan H., *Monosodium L-Glutamate: Its Pharmacology and Role in the Chinese Restaurant Syndrome* (Science, Vol. 163, 1969)

(86) Selby, George, and Lance, James W., *Observations on 500 Cases of Migraine and Allied Vascular Headache* (Journal of Neurology, Neurosurgery and Psychiatry, Vol. 23, 1960)

(87) Shanbrom, E., *Treatment of Herpetic Pain and Post-Herpetic Neuralgia with Intravenous Procaine* (Journal of the American Medical Association, Vol. 176, 1961)

(88) Sicuteri, Federigo, *Mast Cells and Their Active Substances. Their Role in the Pathogenesis of Migraine* (Headache, Vol. 3, 1963)

(89) Sicuteri, Federigo, *Vasoneuroactive Substances and Their Implication in Vascular Pain* in Research and Clinical Studies in Headache (Basel, New York: Karger, Vol. 1, 1967)

(90) Sicuteri, Federigo, *The Ingestion of Serotonin Precursors (L-5-hydroxytryptophan and L-tryptophan) Improves Migraine Headache* (Headache, Vol. 13, 1973)

(91) Sicuteri, Federigo, *Headache as Possible Expression of Deficiency of Brain 5-hydroxytryptamine (Central Denervation Supersensitivity* (Headache, Vol. 14, 1974)

(92) Sigerist, H.E., *A History of Medicine. Vol. 1. Primitive and Archaic Medicine* (New York: Oxford University Press, 1955)

(93) Skinhøj, Erik, *Hemodynamic Studies Within the Brain During Migraine* (Archives of Neurology, Vol. 29, 1973)

(94) Somerville, Brian W., *The Role of Progesterone in Menstrual Migraine* (Neurology, Minneapolis, Vol. 21, 1971)

(95) Somerville, Brian W., *The Role of Estradiol Withdrawal in the Etiology of Menstrual Migraine* (Neurology, Minneapolis, Vol. 22, 1972)

(96) Sulman, F.G., *Serotonin-Migraine in Climatic Heat Stress, Its Prophylaxis and Treatment.* Proceedings of the International Headache Symposium, Elsinore, Denmark, 1971 (Basle: Sandoz Ltd., 1971)

(97) Sulman, F.G., Danon, A., Pfeifer, Y., Tal, E., and Weller, C.P., *Urinal-ysis of Patients Suffering from Climatic Heat Stress (Sharav)* (International Journal of Biometeorology, Vol. 14, 1970)

(98) Symonds, Charles P., *Cough Headache* (Brain, Vol. 79, 1956)

(99) Taylor, Alex R., *Post-Concussional Sequelae* (British Medical Journal, Vol. 2, 1967)

(100) Trewethie, E.R., and Khaled, L., *Wine and Migrainous Neuralgia* (British Medical Journal, Vol. 1, 1972)

(101) Tubbs, O.N., and Potter, J.M., *Early Post-Concussional Headache* (Lancet, Vol. 2, 1970)

(102) Von Klein, C.H., *The Medical Features of the Papyrus Ebers* (Journal of the American Medical Association, Vol. 45, 1905)

(103) Walshe, Sir Francis, *Head Injuries as a Factor in the Aetiology of Intracranial Meningioma* (Lancet, Vol. 2, 1961)

(104) Warner, G., and Lance, J.W., *Relaxation Therapy in Migraine and Chronic Tension Headache* (Medical Journal of Australia, Vol. 1, 1975)

(105) Waters, W.E., and O'Connor, P.J., *The Clinical Validation of a Head-ache Questionnaire* in *Background to Migraine, Third British Migraine Symposium* (London: Heinemann, 1970)

(106) Weiss, Edward, and English, O. Spurgeon, *Psychosomatic Medicine* (Philadelphia, London; W.B. Saunders, 1957)

(107) Whitty, C.W.M., and Hockaday, J.M., *Migraine. A Follow-up Study of 92 Patients* (British Medical Journal, Vol. 1, 1968)

(108) Wolff, Harold G., *Headache and Other Head Pain* (New York: Oxford University Press, 1963)

Notes

CHAPTER 1

Page 4
The quotation from the Ebers Papyrus is from the translation by W.R. Dawson cited by Sigerist [92] p. 340. The explanatory brackets (castor oil plant) have been added by the author. Further information about this important papyrus may be found in [65] p. 547 and [102] p. 1928.
Doctor Henry Ernest Sigerist occupied Chairs in The History of Medicine in Leipzig, and Johns Hopkins, Baltimore, then became Research Associate in the History of Medicine at Yale University.
Babylonian poem cited by [69] p. 6 and [92] p. 451.

Page 6
The cure of Case number 29 at Epidaurus is quoted by Douglas Guthrie, Medical Historian of Edinburgh. [42] p. 44.
The description of migraine by Hippocrates is quoted by Dr. Macdonald Critchley [23] p. 28.

Page 7
Quotation from Aretaeus [2] p. 294.

Page 8
Quotation from Paul of Aegina [1] p. 350
Quotation from Willis cited by Critchley [23] p. 33.

Page 10
Cherokee ritual quoted by Sigerist [92] p. 205.

Pages 11–12
For Pickering's work on histamine headache see [79] p. 77.
Harold G. Wolff's book is reference [109].
The story of George Bernard Shaw is told by Lennox and Lennox [63] p. 438.

CHAPTER 2

Pages 15–16
Information on pain threshold from [108] p. 12.
One of the Aphorisms of Hippocrates [3] p. 298.

Page 20
Quotation from "The Ice-Cream Headache" [52] p. 236.
Daniel Drake is quoted in the *Journal of the Royal College of Physicians of London*, Vol. 6, No. 3, 1972, p. 328. The full title of his book is given in [26].

Page 22
The information concerning "hot-dog" headaches is taken from [46] p. 1162.

Page 23
Studies on Chinese Restaurant Syndrome in [85] p. 826.

Page 24
Reports of histamine content in alcoholic drinks came from references [41] p. 1320, [75] p. 241 and [100] p. 290. Doctor Trewethie has supplied further information to me by letter. Doctor Ough quotes other studies in which up to 30 mg/litre of histamine has been found in some red wines, particularly those from the Burgundy district of France.

Pages 27–28
Reports on cough headache in references [98] p. 557 and [83] p. 801.

Page 28
The quotation from Hippocrates is in [3] p. 94, but italics have been added by the author.
Harold G. Wolff refers to the subject in [108] p. 493–4.

Page 29
Description of my own patients with benign sex headache will be found in [57].

Page 30
Data from Masters and Johnson [67] p. 278, p. 294 and following pages.

Page 31
Doctors Paulson and Klawans' report will be found in [76] p. 181.

CHAPTER 3

Page 34
Doctor Kerr's hypothesis is put forward in [53] p. 168.
Doctor Jannetta's observations are contained in [51].

Page 37
The use of cortisone for the prevention of pain in shingles is described by Dr. F.A.Elliott of Philadelphia [31] p. 610.
The place of the intravenous administration of local anesthetic agents in the management of post-herpetic neuralgia is discussed by Dr. Edward Shanbrom [87] p. 1041.

Page 43
Costen's Syndrome is named after Dr. James B. Costen of the Department of Otolaryngology, Washington University School of Medicine, St. Louis, who first described it [22] p. 1.

CHAPTER 4

Page 57
Vitamin A intoxication in the Antarctic expedition is discussed in [21] p. 1337.

Page 60
The relationship of headache to blood pressure is covered in [108] p. 476 and following pages.

Page 65
Extracts from Kingsford Smith's diary taken from Ward McNally's book *Smithy* [70] p. 99–101.

Page 68
Quotation from Hippocrates [3] p. 54.

CHAPTER 5

Page 73
The estimate of 1 in 2000 for tumors of the nervous system is made from statistics in [15] p. 1.

Page 81
A brief history of the development of the new X-ray technique is given in an Editorial entitled "Computer Assisted Tomography" in *The British Medical Journal*, Vol. 1 (June 22), 1974, p. 623.

CHAPTER 6

Page 88
Doctor Brenner and his colleagues described their work in [14] p. 379.

Page 89
The study from Oxford, England, is reported in [101] p. 128.

Pages 89–90
The treatment regime used in Helsinki, Finland, is described in [81] p. 777.

Page 91
Doctor Wolff's opinions are expressed in [108] p. 617 and following pages.

Page 93
Doctor Cyriax's views will be found in [24] p. 193.

Page 94
Doctor Wolff's study of muscle contraction as a cause of post-traumatic headache is in [108] p. 618 and following.

Page 95
Cushing's figures are cited by Sir Francis Walshe in the paper from which he is quoted [103] p. 993.

Pages 95–96
Doctors Balla and Moraitis' conclusions are from [8] p. 355.

Page 96
Doctor Ellard's observations are in [30] p. 349.

Pages 97–98
Doctor Taylor is quoted from [99] p. 67.

Page 98
Professor Miller is quoted from [71] p. 919 and p. 992.

Page 99
Reference to Ellard [30] p. 349.

CHAPTER 7

Page 103
Clinic statistics from [61] p. 909.

Page 105
Tweedledum and Tweedledee are quoted from Chapter 4 of Lewis Carroll's *Through the Looking Glass* [19].

Page 107
Doctor Wolff's studies on tension headache [108] p. 582.

Page 108
Family history of headache from [36] p. 773.

Page 109
Doctor Every has not yet published his work in detail but a brief account will be found in [33] p. 37, and in *The Lancet* of March 27, 1965, p. 685.

Page 110
The conclusions of Friedman and his colleagues are based on a study of 2000 patients [36] p. 773.
Mayo Clinic report is [66] p. 184.

Page 112
Weiss and English [106] have sections on headache (p. 445) and migraine (p. 453). Treatment suggestions are quoted from the latter.

Pages 113–14
See Jacobsen's book [50]. For results of relaxation therapy in headache see [9] p. 49 and [104] p. 298.

CHAPTER 8

Page 123
Doctor Erik Skinhøj injected a radioactive isotope into the internal carotid artery of patients with classic and common migraine and found that blood flow increased in both forms during the headache phase. Flow was diminished in "classic migraine" while neurological symptoms were being experienced. Chemical changes in the cerebro spinal fluid in both forms of migraine showed that parts of the brain had been deprived of oxygen at some stage of the migraine attack [93] p. 95.

Pages 124–25
Quotations in this chapter from authors in the eighteenth and nineteenth centuries are taken from Liveing [64].

Page 126
The Cheshire Cat is found in Chapter 6 of Lewis Carroll's *Alice in Wonderland* [17].

Page 128
Description of basilar artery migraine by Bickerstaff [10] 1057.
Vomiting attacks in childhood are discussed in a clinical study of 500 migrainous patients by Dr. Anthony and myself [58] p. 356.

Page 131
Tissot quoted by Liveing [64].
Fever in migraine, see [84] p. 45 and p. 57.

Page 133
For long-term follow-up of migraine, see [107] p. 735.
Professor Bille's work is reported in [11].

Pages 133–34
Surveys of headache in a biscuit factory [38] p. 44, and in general practice
[20] p. 14.

Page 134
For Professor Bille's study see [11].
Professor Dalsgaard-Nielsen reported his findings in [25] p. 18.

Page 135
Survey of Doctors Waters and O'Connor in [105] p. 1.

CHAPTER 9

Page 137
Professor Bille's studies, see [11]
Doctors Selby and Lance's figures on personality characteristics of migrain-
ous patients taken from [86] p. 23.

Pages 137–38
Study of Doctors Henryk-Gutt and Rees [47] p. 141.
For study of allergy and epilepsy see [58] p. 356.

Page 139
Footballer's migraine, see [68] p. 326.
For migraine following head injuries in children, see [43] p. 548.

Page 140
For effects of changes in barometric pressure see [4] p. 1035, [32] p. 650 and
[54] p. 849.

Page 141
For effect of weather on migraine, see [96], p. 45, and [97] p. 205.

Page 142
The study of Drs. Henryk-Gutt and Rees is reported in [47] p. 141.

Pages 142–43
Labarraque quoted by Liveing [64].

Page 143
Friedman's essay, see [34] p. 661.

Pages 144–45
Studies on REM sleep in [26] p. 513
Galen is quoted by Liveing [64].

Page 146
See Selby and Lance [86] p. 23.
Harold G. Wolff's studies will be found in [108] p. 327.
The London Hospital Study is [74] p. 445.

Page 147
The comparison of tyramine and an inactive substance in the production of migraine is contained in [48] p. 113 and [73] p. 496.

Pages 147–48
The effect of a low blood sugar in precipitating migraine is discussed by Blau and Cumings [12] p. 1242, Blau and Pike [13] p. 241 and Pearce [77] p. 154.

Page 148
Cornelius Celsus is quoted by Critchley [25] p. 28.

Pages 148–49
Edward Liveing [64]. Brackets (of migraine) inserted by author.

Page 150
Lance and Anthony see [58] p. 356.
Doctor Somerville's work is reported in [94] p. 853 and [95] p. 355.

Page 152
Quote from Dr. Friedman [35] p. 165.

CHAPTER 10

Page 153
Möllendorf quoted by Liveing [64]
Quotation from Critchley [23] p. 28.

Page 154
Darwin quoted by Harold G. Wolff [108] p. 259–265.
Observations on pain from scalp arteries in [80] p. 813.

Page 155
Wolff's observations on "neurokinin," a substance like bradykinin [108] p. 319.
Pain produced by serotonin and bradykinin [89] p. 6.

Pages 155–56
Goltman's observations [40] p. 351.

Page 156
Studies of cerebral blood flow by Skinhøj [93] p. 95.

Page 157
Lashley's personal observations in [62] p. 331.

Page 158
Hubel and Wiesel's experiments [49] p. 215.

Pages 158–59
Brindley and Lewin's experiments [16] p. 479.

Page 159
Quotation from Canto No. 4 of *Rape of the Lock*, by Alexander Pope [79] lines 22–24.

Page 160
Sicuteri's hypothesis is put forward in [90] p. 19 and [91]

Page 164
The relationship of serotonin to migraine is summarized in [5] p. 29.

Pages 164–65
The use of the serotonin precursor (5-hydroxytryptophan) in treatment is described by Sicuteri [90] p. 19, and treatment with MAO inhibitors is described in [6] p. 263.

Page 165
Effects of prostaglandin E_1 in normal subjects [17] p. 423.

Pages 166–67
Discussion of mast cells found in [88] p. 86.

CHAPTER 11

Page 172
Psychological treatment of migraine reported in [72] p. 137.
The results of relaxation therapy in our own clinic are reported in [104] and the benefits of transcendental meditation in [9] p. 49.

Page 176
Doctor James Cyriax is quoted from [24] p. 139.

Pages 177–78
For results of intravenous histamine drip, see [86] p. 23.

CHAPTER 12

Page 188
Romberg's original description of cluster headache is in [82] p. 56.

Pages 188–89
Harris's description is amplified in [45] p. 457.

Page 189
For the work of Horton and his colleagues, see [48] p. 257.
Blood histamine in cluster headache [7] p. 225.
Paper by Dr. Kunkle and his colleagues in [55] p. 510.
Clinical description based on a series of 60 patients reported by myself and Dr. Anthony [60] p. 401.

Page 191
Doctor Ekbom presents some aspects of his detailed clinical study of cluster headache in [29] p. 176.
Doctor Graham's recent observations on cluster headache are contained in [40] p. 175.

Page 193
Doctor Horton's observations on skin temperature [48] p. 257.
Our own thermographic studies are described in [59], p. 240 and in my book [56] p. 163 and plate 1. Those of Dr. Friedman and his associates are in [37] p. 1.
Arteriographic study of Drs. Ekbom and Greitz [28] p. 1.

Pages 195–96
Romberg's quotation from [82] p. 57.

Index

229